THE BUSY KID

MY BIPOLAR JOURNEY

DANA WALL

CONTENTS

FOREWORD

As a man in America, speaking out about mental health problems and treatment represents a huge act of bravery. Even as scientists make strides toward understanding the causes of mental health disorders and how best to treat them, the social stigma around psychiatric diagnosis and treatment often prevents people suffering from mental illness from seeking treatment (Parcesepe & Cabassa, 2013). Although mental health stigma has far reaching consequences for all of us, these problems seem to be worse for men, who are much less likely than women to seek needed mental health treatment (Sagar-Ouriaghli et al., 2019). In this book, a man with serious mental health symptoms finds the courage to stand up and tell his story.

As the beloved teacher of my secondary school choir class for six years, Dana Wall told us a lot of stories. Much like those in this book, they often tackled serious content with a quirky sense of humor and an inspirational tone. Sitting on that conductor's podium, he directed our voices-- but he also encouraged and inspired us. He used his stories to convey wisdom, and to let us know that he cared for and was proud of us.

Now it's my turn to be proud of him. By telling his story in living, unapologetic color, he is able to buck the typical pattern in which men with mental illness hide their stories due to fear of judgment (or possible discrimination). In a culture that glorifies some imagined ideal of stoicism and stability in men, sharing in this way takes a lot of courage. My hope is that other men will read these stories and realize that they, too, can come out of the proverbial shadows and get help, perhaps with a little less fear of being judged or stigmatized for doing so.

In this book, Wall describes his symptoms of bipolar disorder over the course of his life, his decision to seek help, and his ongoing work in treatment. He shares his experiences coming to terms with diagnosis, as well as his experiences in psychotherapy and taking medications. Beyond these details, Wall uses narrative to illustrate a tug-of-war that will resonate with many people who have experienced bipolar disorder: On the one hand, can I affirm and honor my psychological differences (for example, being a person who has intense positive emotions and spontaneity) as a good and interesting part of who I am? But on the other hand, can I also acknowledge that I need treatment so that these differences do not become extreme and cause problems? It's easy to cling to one or the other, but much harder to hold both of these truths at the same time. Wall emerges from these pages as a whole person rather than a diagnosis, gently holding both his vulnerability and his pride without diluting either one.

May his act of bravery inspire us all to share our own stories.

Tory Eisenlohr-Moul, Ph.D

Clinical Psychologist

Assistant Professor of Psychiatry

University of Illinois at Chicago

Mr Wall's Concert Choir Class of 2004

INTRODUCTION

I'm not a doctor. I'm not a psychiatrist, psychologist, counselor, or specialist of any kind. But over the years, I've been through the office doors of all of them countless times trying to sort out my life and make sense of a sickness that has been difficult to understand. To say I succeeded would be a lie. To say I've had failures and successes would be more accurate. I haven't lived forever, but statistics have put me in a good slot compared to the millions of people on the globe who have suffered with bipolar disorder. I've read, listened, and learned as much as I could about people who have struggled with mania and depression, as I have, and decided that if anyone can benefit from hearing my story then I have an obligation to tell it.

As one flips through the following pages, there may be some things they don't want to read. It is hoped this isn't an excuse to put the book down. Nobody wanted to hear they should wear their seatbelt in the early 70s, but it turned out to be a pretty good idea. There might be something hiding within the pages of this book that is useful, as well. When first diagnosed with bipolar disorder, I struggled with listening to people tell me I had it. I slowly learned to cope with it. Within this writing, I would like to describe how bipolar disorder changed my life.

There is a reason behind the title "The Busy Kid." For three decades, "busy kid" best described me. As a child, I could create or recreate most anything with a good sharp pencil. I drew pictures around the clock, creating stories and cartoons whenever I could. School seemed to be a good place to do a little extra drawing. It didn't take long to finish my schoolwork, after which I would continue drawing. I remember the teacher saying to me, "Dana, you're not holding your pencil correctly. That's okay for drawing, but for writing you should hold it like this." Oddly, my penmanship seemed to look as good as everyone else's even though I allegedly didn't know how to hold my damned pencil.

I never understood why everyone else went to bed so early. If I went to bed at midnight, I woke up at two thinking about a current project or I wrote a song. I often woke up at five-thirty or earlier while other people slept until eight. As a kid, sleeping at someone else's house, I remember lying there with a million ideas in my head for what seemed like hours, waiting for my friend to wake up. After I became an adult, I would often pull a twenty-hour day. I put notepads by my bedside to write things down in, lying there awake with ideas scurrying around in my brain. Why didn't other people do that? How come when I walked outside at two in the morning, the only light in the neighborhood came from my house? It couldn't be important. I'd been running in high gear all of my life and sometimes would go for days without shutting off at all. What I always knew, but hadn't taken into account, is there can't be a top without a bottom, an in without an out, a back without a front....or an up without a down. Down was sure to come. I just didn't know it yet.

STARING AT THE WALLS

atching four children play on a swing set is one of the little things. The little things warm our hearts and make the world a better place. Just about every day in the 60s, we would run out to the swingset with the wind in our hair and bring all that metal to life. Our little hands would grip firmly on the chains as we pumped our legs back and forth, reaching out to the sky. Sounds of laughter rang through the air. Today would not be an ordinary day in our backyard.

We were delighted as Dad ran out to play on the swing set for the first time. We grinned from ear to ear, wondering where he would go first. Would he go to the glider or the swings? Maybe he'd go to one of the bars at the end and climb high to the top as the older children often did. But he set his sights on the slide. He didn't climb the ladder, though. He came armed with car wax and polished the shiny silver slide, buffing it with vigor. We figured out his plan when he finished and one of the kids climbed to the top of the ladder. We'd never gone so fast! For the rest of the afternoon, we took turns flying down the slide and for some reason, with each trip down it seemed to go faster. We polished it with our bottoms a little more every time we slid down. However, Dad had a different motive.

Later in the afternoon, the '61 Falcon station wagon pulled into the driveway. Mom came home from work and would slide down the slide as she did almost every day. For some reason, Dad couldn't be found. If we thought about it, we could have seen him peering from one of the windows inside of the house. Mom climbed to the top of the ladder and exclaimed "Look at me! Look at me!" All eyes were on her as she gave herself a shove and began her voyage to the bottom of the slide. She traveled downward at an alarming speed with her skirt up over her head and her arms flailing. Her feet were up a little higher than other times and if one listened closely, they would hear her shrill scream. Car wax must be one of the little things too. Dad used just a little of it and all four of us got a lot of enjoyment out of it. It enhanced Mom's trip down the slide as well. But the truth is, Dad got more enjoyment out of the car wax than anyone.

As the youngest of four children, I took my share of teasing and caught my share of the hell growing up with an older brother and two older sisters. We spent a lot of time playing outside in the woods and hills surrounding our home. We lived in a beautiful three-bedroom house my Dad built from the ground up, and survived a tragedy there. In November of 1963 it burned to the ground. A year later we moved into a new home my Dad built on the same foundation. It set us back, but I'm sure it helped make our family foundation even stronger than the one my father built our home on.

During the time of his thirty-seven-year career, phones were installed in people's homes. Telephone lines were up on poles and they needed good men to climb up and work on them. They needed men to service the lines that went into homes and check for trouble. They needed men to add multiple lines to homes and put up with cranky people who wanted things their way. That's where my Dad came in. Being smart and funny and good at his job, he knew how to deal with those cranky people and could talk them down when needed.

He hurt his back climbing telephone poles in his thirties and from then on, he walked a little slower and tolerated a lot of pain. This may be why we loved him and feared him at the same time. Very firm and often fair, he liked to have fun with us, but didn't put up with any shit. He liked to play basketball with us, throw snowballs, and get down on the floor and wrestle when he could. He loved playing with us but expected us to follow certain rules.

Sometimes he made things up as he went. Dad's rules were vague. With Dad, the rules were not discussed very often but we all knew where we stood. We all held jobs, worked for our money, paid for our own cars, and lived by curfews. If we came in late we would see him standing in front of the picture window big as a giant as we drove up the driveway. If that happened, we knew we were in trouble. I'm not sure of my own take on it, be it "Follow the rules" or "Don't get caught!" But I knew Dad cared about us. He nurtured us and taught us, but he didn't do any of it alone.

My Mom might be the original multi-tasker. She could work miracles. For most of my young life she worked as a secretary. She had sharp organizational skills because of it. She took care of all of us, held a full time job, belonged to a service club (which she still belongs to) and found time to go to church, give to the poor, and take care of the household. Mom would buzz around the kitchen making freezer jam early in the morning before work. She made her own sweet relish, canned peaches, froze corn, made ground bologna, and much more. Fast food didn't happen around our house. She served good homemade food even though she worked every day. She kept lists to help organize all of her activities, including holidays. She kept track of meals, gifts and greeting cards. I don't know when she slept, but she got everything done and started over the next day.

In 1971 we got a call from a far away relative. Because he didn't call very often, it must've been important. This call would change all of our lives. My uncle struggled with alcoholism while going through a divorce with an alcoholic woman. They could no longer take care of their four-year-old son. After a lot of discussion and a great deal of thought, my parents decided to take the young boy into our home. I think a lot of this decision fell on my Mom. She would never deny a young child the chance at a better life. And that's what Erik got. He came into a warm, clean, caring home all because of Mom. She provided for him just as she provided for all of us and he soon stopped referring to her as his aunt and started calling her "Mom."

I didn't know my older brother, Daryl, very well growing up. Because of an eight year age gap, we weren't always very close. In high school, his athletic skills were amazing. I looked up to him for this ability, as did everyone else, and when I got older, people compared us. I didn't possess any of his athletic ability. I felt as though I lived in his shadow a lot. But when I grew older something good happened. Daryl bought my Grandpa's farm right next door. At the time I didn't think much of it, but this would be the way I would build a relationship with my big brother. I learned to laugh, drink, tell stories, and do all the things that were missing from my relationship with my older brother. It wouldn't be long and he'd give me an unforgettable gift.

The night before my wedding, Daryl and I got pretty hammered. I didn't think I'd remember any of it. It turned out to be a night I'd never forget. My brother took me into his hotel room and started talking to me, almost in tears. He gave me a small wooden box. A beautiful pocket-watch that once belonged to my Grandfather beamed from inside. My Grandfather gave it to him hoping he could one day pass it on to his son. Daryl told me he would never have children and wanted me to pass it on to my son one day. I grew closer to my brother that night than ever before. To this day we're close brothers and close friends; he's one of three people who mean more to me than anyone in the world.

My oldest sister, Toni, could do most anything. Why did God give her all the talent? She could draw and paint. She could play the piano and guitar. She could ride a unicycle and run like the wind. She had a beautiful singing voice. Patience, humor and intelligence were all rolled up into one beautiful package. I never understood why someone with all of these wonderful talents and "features" would be here for such a short time. Why would she get the rug pulled out from under her the way she did? Multiple Sclerosis set in when she was about thirty. After she started having children, she started getting tingling sensations, which would later turn to numbing sensations, thus beginning *her* life journey.

The girl who could perform the Chinese splits and ride a unicycle for miles started to weaken. Multiple Sclerosis caused her to be unsteady on her feet. She would often attend sporting events at the school as her husband was the superintendent. Because she often stumbled, people started rumors that she drank. It embarrassed her enough that she started using a cane to get people to stop talking about her. Later she moved to a wheelchair where she would spend the rest of her life. I can't be sure, but I think she spent about twelve years in that damned chair. Calmness, patience, and passiveness helped her survive the personal hell she had there, but at just fifty-three years old she left the earth and went to a better place. Every time I dream about her, (which is quite often) I see her walking. It makes me feel good to know she's walking in the kingdom of God.

When my youngest sister, Nikki, enters the room, people notice. It has always been that way. She's cute, fun, and wonderful to be around. She dresses to her full potential at all times and treats people the way they want to be treated. A lot of people think about things they'd like to do and have dreams they'd like to accomplish. My sister does them. She's a military mom and goes above and beyond the call of duty to support not just her own son, but as many young men and women who give their lives to their country as she can. It doesn't stop there.

She decided to help the people in her community at Christmastime. She dressed up as Mrs. Claus and went to medical care facilities and preschools to conduct sing-a-longs for the elderly people and young children she met along the way. She made a dress and got a wig and glasses and developed a song list. The community loved the idea and her schedule filled right up. Soon Mrs. Claus became a celebrity in her small town. She's a caring person with the ideas and energy to make people happy. But this is just one of the many charity events she's involved herself in. Somehow she's found a way to do several of them, and the world is a better place because of her.

Sometimes it's good for a family to be shaken up a little bit. That's what happened when my soon to be younger brother, Erik, arrived. A four-year-old can bring challenges to a home. We didn't know it at first, but fetal alcohol syndrome would be one of our biggest challenges. A lot of personal and social problems came into his life and he had difficulty dealing with them. As a child, and also later in his life, he would often be destructive, taking things apart that he couldn't put back together. Very often, things would end up broken with no explanation. Although troubled, he brought humor and charm to the family. As time went on I stopped referring to him as my cousin and started calling him my brother. That's what he would be for the rest of his life. When he got older, he married and his children arrived. He and his wife were later separated and it became too much for him. Depression got the best of him and he took his own life before his twenty-sixth birthday. We suffered with this loss for years. As with any devastating news, it left a hard healing mark on us. For me, it triggered emotions I'd never felt before. But in time, we were able to move on with our lives. We dusted ourselves off and forged ahead the best we could.

As for me, the youngest of four, I never felt that I fit in. There were too many things to accomplish and not enough hours in the day. I lived in the shadow of older siblings who were bright, beautiful, talented, and athletic. I saw myself as none of those things. In my own mind, I felt like the black sheep of the family. I never felt smart, considered myself ugly compared to my siblings, and was seldom satisfied with what I created. Being uncoordinated put me at a disadvantage when others made athletics look easy. I often had trouble explaining ideas when the thoughts in my head seemed clear. But yet, I was the "busy kid." I had just a little bit too much energy. Where did I come from and where would I go? With a pencil in my hand and a million ideas in my head, what would I come up with next?

2

BUSY OR NOT, HERE I COME!

I pulled the cord, lowered the ladder, and peered into the dark, spooky attic. Once inside, I screwed in the dusty, cold light bulb and lit the area holding my Tyco Race Track. It rained buckets today, making it a perfect time to sprawl miniature miles of track all over the dining room table. While I scurried around the attic looking for the box with all of the cars and track pieces that would bring the table to life, I found all kinds of other treasures. Wooden blocks, army men, cardboard, and a big paper tube from the center of a roll of wrapping paper were just a few of the things I would use to spice up my creation. When I returned to the main floor dining room, or "control center," I started to build the racetrack, hoping it would be my workplace for the next few days.

There were many decisions to be made when laying out the design for my track. How long would each straight stretch be? How much slope could I put in it and still get maximum speed? How tight should I make the corners so the cars wouldn't always fall off of the track?

It didn't stop there. Should I make buildings out of paper to represent the pit stop, concession stand, etc.? Or did I want to build an entire town? An entire town would be more challenging, so it won the debate. Houses, a library, a school, a store, and just about anything else I could think of would be built out of blocks, boxes, paper, or whatever I could find. I would need a parking lot with personalized parking spaces for all of the cars, because someone I knew drove them. But the process still didn't stop.

I built a service station, because anyone with a toy racetrack knows that the cars often needed to be taken apart to have the contacts cleaned, as well as the brushes and magnets. I enjoyed cleaning and repairing the cars as they rolled into the service station. For an eight-year-old with a little imagination, this meant I could talk to customers as they came into the garage, work on cars, take them for test drives, and return them to their rightful owners. I might spend a whole day talking to myself and getting all of the cars in working order.

A grandstand made of cardboard with a hand-drawn audience surrounded the track. The American flag would fly proudly against the sky and the National Anthem would be sung before each race. What started out as a simple day became a week of hard work and creativity. Each night when I went to bed, I would lie awake thinking of ways to improve upon my design and consider new things to build. The dining room table donned a racetrack and a rather large, always-growing town made of paper, wooden blocks, little plastic army men and other random toys and junk. What started out as "Mom, can I play with my racetrack today?" turned out to be "Mom, can I build a large three-dimensional project on your dining room table that will be there over a week and take two days to tear down?" Not being one to stifle creativity, Mom let me borrow the dining room table for a while.

When you're a kid, you're a kid. That's all there is to it. In the 60s people weren't often labeled or diagnosed. The quiet ones were told to speak up. The loud ones were told to shut up. For most little kids, life went smoothly. We got up, went to school, went home, played for a while, did our homework, and went to bed. The process soon started over. But for a lot of kids, having recess at school and time to play at home didn't burn off all the energy they had inside. Or maybe a million ideas scurried in their heads and they felt like they were going to burst. Many kids, including me, were able to find ways to burn off extra energy without getting into too much trouble. But some kids found that acting out worked best. They made a little extra noise.

Now, were they being naughty? Remember, the 60s were upon us. Of course they were being naughty. Today we'd say they were being impulsive. We might say they were having trouble concentrating, or staying on task. But years ago, if a kid didn't stay on task, hold his pencil correctly and do his work, he was naughty. He wrote sentences or stood in the corner. He clapped erasers or put his head down. Today we understand writing to be something students should enjoy. If it's used as punishment, the fun is taken out of it and it becomes work instead of a pleasant way to pass the time. We now know standing in the corner puts a student on a pedestal for what they've done and makes an example of them instead of correcting the real problem. In the 60s, students with extra energy were often called "busy" or "hyper" and were punished for those things. Today, in most cases, the best way to approach the problem is to find out why a kid acts out, does impulsive things, or has trouble staying on task in the first place.

If a math teacher gives story problems and one finds himself wanting to finish writing the story, does that make him naughty? If he has trouble taking multiple choice tests because he can't finish reading all of the choices without losing focus or forgetting which ones said what, does that make him stupid? I think every child has problems like these at one time or another. For some children, it happens on occasion. For others, it happens all day, every day. Some learn how to disguise these issues so they can function "normally" without creating a problem.

As a child, I would often think of some of the things we worked on in school and later do them my own way instead of someone else's. There had to be more than one way to do a story problem, after all.

I often thought of more than one way to do things. My way or someone else's way? My way often won and that didn't make it wrong. Did it? Unfortunately, most adults didn't like it when 8-year-old boys told them they'd found a different way to do something. At least, that's what experience showed me. They seemed happier when students sat at their desk and did the assignment the way they were supposed to with as few questions and as few "suggestions" as possible. But I was a wiggler. I was the one who needed to go to the bathroom, or get a drink all the time as a way to move around, so I wouldn't explode from all of the extra energy. Frequent trips to the pencil sharpener, the water fountain, or bathroom didn't make me all that popular with the teachers.

As a youngster I got up at six in the morning on a Saturday and drew pictures, watching the test pattern on television while waiting for cartoons to start. Then I might go outside and build things, run, and play until dark and then sit up late at night in my room drawing, building with an erector set, or writing stories when I should've been asleep. Because I didn't act out or get into any trouble, no one noticed my insomnia at just eight years old. I did this almost every night. It seemed "normal." People knew of ADHD or Attention Deficit Hyperactive Disorder but didn't often diagnose it. Manic depression (bipolar disorder) was largely ignored. Since I learned to corral my energy and never suffered from depression, I remained a "busy" kid. Since I liked to create, liked music, liked artwork, liked to build, and liked to write, finding things to do came easy. But, as stated earlier, you can't have an up without a down. At some point, going at full speed would catch up with me.

For this young busy kid, life didn't catch up. I needed things to do. I needed ways to stimulate creativity, burn off energy, and keep from getting into trouble. As a youngster, I didn't often get in trouble, but I was frequently misunderstood by adults. I often got confused stares from them as I rattled off a long story or told of an idea I had. In about the sixth grade, I had a teacher who told me I should learn to shut my mind off once in a while. I wasn't sure what that meant, so I continued to do things in the way that came natural to me.

Because we lived in the country, I could go into the woods and find things to do out there. There was a big dump out in the woods behind our house with all kinds of things in it for me to recycle. I would build "Soapbox Derby" type go-karts and ride them down the hills. Not paved hills, mind you. I just rode down hills with dirt, rocks, bushes, all kinds of obstructions. When I got to the bottom, the go-kart would be in pieces, so I would nail it back together, haul it back up the hill and start over. When I got old enough, I started working on mechanized things, like lawnmowers and cars. I always needed something to keep me busy. When friends came over, they acted like they were in a museum or an amusement park. There was always an abundance of new things to see and do.

There were all kinds of "busy" kids. Some were troublemakers who couldn't keep their mouths shut or their hands to themselves. They ran everywhere they went and when they got there, they ran into something. They said inappropriate things, did inappropriate things, and got into a lot of trouble. Another type of "busy" kid ran on full speed most of the time and then, for some reason or another, just kind of slipped out of the picture for a while. They would become withdrawn and no one knew why. If they were asked to come out and do something, they wouldn't. But after a while, they would emerge and start the process all over again.

But possessing "busy" or "hyper" qualities didn't have to mean trouble. For some, it meant productivity. Most of the kids with an extra boost of energy were very creative. They were often the artists, musicians, dancers, writers, and builders, though staying on task until they completed the project or being satisfied with what they produced could be difficult.

For me, the product *never* came out the same as the one in my mind. I could create all kinds of things in my head and when I recreated them on paper or built them, they often turned out beautiful, but not quite the way I envisioned them. The onlooker saw something wonderful, something new and fresh that I created. They would give me praise for what I did and I would smile and say thank you. But, for me, I saw something that didn't measure up to what I had envisioned. I felt as though I took credit for an inferior product. In my own mind, I never quite did what I set out to do. In fact, I felt that I'd failed. Growing up, I felt a lot of failure; but not the same kind that others felt. People didn't say, "This isn't good enough. Do it again!" They accepted my work as good but I didn't. I drifted by, feeling that even though others accepted my work, it was likely substandard.

I dealt with the feeling of failure as I got older as well. As an adult, working as a teacher, I received a lot of positive feedback for the work I did but seldom felt as though I deserved it. I almost always felt as though the concerts I performed could have been better. I seldom felt the students responded to me the way I wanted them to. I felt an overwhelming amount of guilt for accepting credit and compliments for the work I did because I knew I could do better. There were plenty of ideas in my head but I didn't like the way they turned out.

During childhood, I coped with the fact that ideas seemed to be spilling out of my ears.

I even coped with the fact that I didn't learn the way everyone else did. In those days, we were all taught the same way. There were seldom teachers who worked with multiple intelligences or listed five different ways to fulfill the assignment. So, in science class, I would ask Mr. Whiting if I could draw a diagram of the heart for extra credit. I would make bulletin boards in my math class pertaining to long division even though I didn't understand it. Being right-brained, math didn't come easy to me. I didn't know about right and left brain learning, but I adapted.

I did anything I could do to survive the traditional classroom setting and I'm surprised I did. Little did everyone know, including myself, I possessed a very misunderstood mood disorder that would grow into something I would have to deal with and learn to control for the rest of my life. When I grew a little older, I turned into quite a storyteller. I credit this ability to both of my parents and my older brother. They all could tell jokes and stories quite well. I watched and listened as they would "spin yarns," and I would repeat what they said but I would often add my own flair to it. Later on I became a music teacher. I believe much of my success as a teacher pointed toward my ability to tell stories. I often had more than eighty students in each of my classes and they would sit captivated as I told some story I made up about moving the refrigerator, then I would turn it into a lesson about sharpening your memory. As a "busy" kid, my personal experiences were very full and random. Collecting data for stories came easy. As much as I used my own experiences and ideas to tell stories, I also learned from them.

My Mother told me a story once and helped me better understand myself. She grew up in poverty. She told me when she was a little girl, another kid asked if they were poor. She said "I don't know." She never thought about it. She never thought of herself as poor and her Mother never talked about it or complained. For me, this related to being bipolar in the 60s and 70s. At this time in my life, I'd never felt depressed and few people ever pointed out my hyperactivity. Everyone just assumed I ran at high speed.

They knew of my creativity. No one ever made me feel different at this point and I just kept on going. Because I worked hard and didn't misbehave much, no one felt the need to reach out to me. Most people were entertained by the fact that I moved at a faster speed than others. I never thought about whether or not I could keep up the pace. I just kept going.

3

THE UPWARD CLIMB!

I looked up as far as I could see. There were mountains and mountains of rock. I NEEDED to climb up there. I didn't have boots, gloves, rope, or equipment of any kind but excitement flowed through me as I tried to climb the enormous cliff. The more I thought about it, the more excited I got. I looked around and saw no one else. Perfect! There were no parents to tell me I couldn't, no annoying little brother to tell on me, and no cousins to slow me down if they tried coming along. So, off I went.

Having managed to sneak away from my family for a while, I'd found something wonderful to do. I stumbled upon a spectacular wall of rock near Lake Fanny Hooe Campground in the Porcupine Mountains. I couldn't wait to get started. I didn't plan much, but just put my foot on a rock and launched myself up to the next level and kept climbing. Each time I pulled myself up, I got a little more excited and looked for another avenue to climb a little higher up the giant rock formation.

I thought it was amazing! I thought I was amazing! I could feel the blood pumping through my veins and the heart pumping in my chest with every pull and every leap as I continued to do something immensely wonderful, and wrong! I shouldn't have been doing it, but I didn't care. I just felt good, proud, and very much in charge as I climbed higher and higher to the top of the cliff. When I reached the top, I jumped up and down with excitement and threw my hands up in the air like a prizefighter. The moment after I caught my breath, I turned around to look at my accomplishment. I could see miles and miles of trees, rocks and countryside, but the most interesting sight was right at the bottom, where I started.

Busy climbing and focusing on being a superhero, I never once looked back. When I reached the top I noticed my Mom, Dad, little brother, aunt, uncle, and two cousins who had been watching me, at least part of the time. They didn't call out to me, or tell me to come back. I think my Dad knew I would struggle to get back down and wanted to watch me figure it out. I never considered a plan for getting back down. Figuring it out meant being torn up and embarrassed from having to perform the task in front of my whole family. I know my Dad figured it would be a lesson for me. When looking back on things and realizing my manic state during that little "escapade," I'm not sure the lesson stuck. Even though I got all cut up climbing off of the huge pile of rock, I remained high as a kite and part of me never came down.

Living with mania for the first thirty years of my life meant living with a brain that never shut off and a scrawny little body to house any of the "activities" the brain could think of. Remembering childhood, I felt nothing bad could ever happen to me. I rounded up a group of young friends who felt the same way or close to it, and if they didn't, they were more than willing to watch me create things and take risks that would make our lives a little more interesting.

The risk taking started out small. Like every kid, I loved riding no-handed and taking my bike over ramps. I liked hearing the dirt rumble underneath my tires and I *loved* the rush I got when the wheels left the earth for a second and I became airborne. When the bike tires made contact with the ramp on the other side, I felt a sense of accomplishment. When they didn't, I picked myself up, dusted myself off, and figured out another way to make the jump. The ramps started to get higher and spaced further apart, though, and it seemed as though my little band of heroes grew smaller.

When I became old enough to drive, I wanted to try out some of the things I'd seen watching "Rockford Files" and some of the other action type television shows. In the 1970's, just about all cars were rear wheel drive, making them perfect for spinning donuts, doing what we called "power-slides", and peeling out. Because my Father ran a pretty tight ship at home and I didn't want to run the risk of being caught dare-deviling in my car, I made sure to go out on back roads and kept my pit crew small.

Bill, Dale, and I would go out on those roads and put

my poor car through hell. But the real adventure began when I noticed a luggage rack on top of the '72 Buick Century wagon belonging to Dale's mother. In those days, the Century wagon, with a good sized V8 engine in it, could suck up pavement without much effort. Dale would be driving down those winding back roads, going like hell, with Bill hanging out the window yelling and screaming. I dove into the excitement mightily. Riding on top of the luggage rack, I held on for dear life, adrenaline coursing through my veins. Many things come back to me as I recall those wild rides, but what I don't remember is being scared. How come I could ride on top of a car with a giant V8 in it, going sixty or seventy miles an hour down a paved road with an inexperienced driver at the wheel and not be utterly terrified? Instead, I enjoyed every minute of it. I often accomplished these feats without fear.

For instance, I saw a friend of mine not long ago, and he reminded me of something I used to do when driving on curvy roads at night. I'd forgotten about it. He said it would scare the daylights out of him, but he never said anything. When approaching a curve, I would shut off my headlights so I could look for oncoming cars. I'd then turn the lights back on. With the road clear, I could swing wider on the curve and go faster around it. After Phil reminded me of this, I recalled how my heart would pump hard in my chest while the lights were out and the thrill I got as I sped through those corners. I loved to drive through the curves a little faster, and since I didn't know fear, I figured no one else in the car did either. I was wrong, of course.

Since movie theatres and bowling alleys weren't on every street corner in the small northwestern Michigan village of Onekama, where I grew up, I found other things to do with my time. Apple orchards painted the skyline and were just the sort of place for us to frolic. Quite often after dark, I would take my car into the orchards with a few friends and fill the back of it up with as many apples as possible. We would spend the rest of the night chucking apples at mailboxes, road signs, people, and anything else that came along the way. I found that a "wrist rocket" could get a small apple to go quite far and became good at driving and firing apples at the same time. None of this is something I'm proud of, but it does show what a decent kid from a good family can do when he's manic all of the time.

I steered clear of the "party" crowd in high school, because I knew if my Dad ever found out, there would be hell to pay. That didn't mean I was free of "substances" however. I smoked quite a bit of pot. I was probably self-medicating and didn't even know it. When I went off to college, abusing alcohol and other stimulants without getting caught by my parents became easier. I felt normal because a lot of my college friends were partying right along with me. However, because I partied more than at night and on weekends, I'm sure I was self-medicating. I still got to class every day and made pretty good grades, but I did enjoy partying and got hammered a lot.

Not long ago, a friend of mine got into a lot of trouble

for drinking and driving. It set me to thinking about my own past and I realized how lucky I've been. I'm sure most people who drink have driven under the influence at one time or another, so if they're smart enough not to do it anymore, they're still very lucky. That's how I feel. I feel fortunate nothing ever happened to me or to anyone else involved in my reckless decisions. I remember on more than one occasion, opening the car door while driving, hanging my head out the door, and throwing up on the ground. I didn't bother to pull over and just kept driving down the road. Mania, binge drinking, and poor decision making led me to do that, I'm sure. Regardless of the reason, I've since recalled that none of my friends ever put me in this position, though I had no qualms doing it to them.

Mania seemed to control my life, though I didn't understand what was happening. High energy levels got me up early. I could work all day, party most of the night, and get by with very little sleep. I think a euphoric state kept me active and energetic. From age sixteen to around twenty-eight years old, things were good. People were flocking into my social scene to enjoy the activities. I'd do most anything for anyone and they knew it.

I'm not sure euphoria is always a good thing, however. I felt wonderful and creative. I went about life anxiously thinking of something to do next, and was always willing to help a friend. I'm sure now that I didn't always make the right decisions when in a manic state. I quite often got carried away, partying and drinking too much. This often put me in situations I shouldn't have been in. I would drink and drive, sometimes become destructive, or say and do things that crossed the line with my friends. I would frequently do things first and consider the outcome later.

I couldn't always concentrate on tasks and often thought beyond conversations. Sometimes while talking, I would look through people. Ideas were sprinting through my head along with thoughts of something I'd get to do as soon as that dreadful conversation ended. I would often interrupt people while they were talking and say whatever impulsive thought I had. Many of these things still happen from time to time, even with medication in place. Through the years I have made a lot of effort to be sensitive to other people and try not to dominate conversations when I become manic or have thoughts other than those that pertain to the conversation at hand. If I keep the ramps at a reasonable height, maybe people will continue to jump them with me.

4

WHAT'S NORMAL ANYWAY?

*T*he morning came and I felt a tickle on my face as I woke up. Soon the sensation grew stronger and I saw my Dad hovering over me with a grin on his face. It was early on a Saturday, and we would soon be leaving to take his '59 Willys Jeep on a camping trip up north. This would be the first time we'd ever done anything like this, just the two of us. I looked forward to it. With the jeep full of food, pop, inflatable mattresses, my tent, and sleeping bags, we were ready for an overnight trip. We set out on US-31 for a wonderful adventure up to some property my uncle owned.

Anyone who's ever ridden in a Willys Jeep understands that they're not built for speed. We crept along the highway for a while when Dad suddenly pulled over. He reached in the back and got out a can of beans and a can of hash, securing them on the exhaust manifold under the hood and continued driving. We drove another forty-five minutes or so and found a picnic table at the side of the road. He took the canned goods off the exhaust manifold and treated us to a nice hot meal. After eating, we continued our journey north along the roads of northern Michigan, enjoying the scenery and conversation we seldom shared together.

When we got to the property, we found ourselves alone. We weren't looking for company, so it didn't bother us and we made camp at the top of a hill. We soon set off to enjoy Sleeping Bear Dunes just a few miles away. We climbed to the top of the dunes and ran back down just like the other people who were enjoying the sand that day. We went on a dune ride where we learned the history of the dunes, then slurped down ice cream on our way back to the campsite. Once back at camp, we lit a fire and decided on what to create for our evening meal. We chose hotdogs, burned to a crisp and swallowed nearly whole.

We retired to our tent for the evening, and were relaxed when a rumbling sound began to shake the earth. Being all of twelve years old, I knew the sound quite well. "Sounds like it's gonna rain, Dad." It did rain. It rained and rained. The walls of the tent blew from side to side as the storm got stronger. My Dad's air mattress sprung a leak so he kept his mouth on the nozzle most of the night. But the tent didn't leak. When we woke up, we found the entire camp wet except for the clothes we slept in. We packed up a wet camp and began driving home. But things were just beginning to get interesting.

We set out on the road and felt a rumble under the wheels of the Jeep and soon found ourselves on the ground changing a tire. Lucky for us, a good spare tire and tools were on board the Willys. I enjoyed working on the Jeep with my Dad. The entire weekend made me feel like just another "normal" little kid.

I've heard it said that "normal is a setting on a washing machine." I've always liked that phrase, because I've often felt if we were to run everyone out of town who wasn't "normal," we'd empty the whole town. I'd even have to grab the seat of my own pants and toss myself out. I'm sure that everyone is different in his or her own way. That's what makes the world spin. That's what makes life interesting, and that's what makes us who we are and gives us individuality. However, if we see someone with one leg, we're quick to point them out as "different." If someone has a skin color unlike everyone else in the area, he or she is singled out. If someone is very short or very tall, we'll often notice the difference. These differences are easy to spot. We just open our eyes and we notice.

But not all differences are easy to see. Some people carry their differences on the inside. To look at them, they seem like everyone else. They have all of their appendages; they walk upright and seem "normal." So what's the problem?

There are several mood disorders that can't be seen. Some people can cover them up, and many can't. Sometimes a mood disorder can be controlled or hidden well for a while, but as the person grows older, the symptoms worsen and he or she can no longer hide the problem. For some people, there are no symptoms at all until later in life. Or perhaps, because they've always gotten along just fine, they've never noticed the symptoms. It's also possible that a treatment hadn't occurred yet, depending on when they were diagnosed. If diagnosed with manic depression, people were sometimes institutionalized, depending on the severity. If not, many people tried to control it on their own. Perhaps they altered their moods with help from friends or family telling them when they needed to adjust their mood swings. They may also have self medicated with tobacco, alcohol, or other stimulants. Remember, bipolar disorder worsens as one grows older, so for many, problems don't occur until later in life.

I felt, for the most part, like everyone else. I grew up with an older brother and two older sisters. My parents were both present in the household. I lived in a small town where everyone knew everyone else and all of their business. The town sat next to a beautiful inland lake in northern Michigan, not far from Lake Michigan. We spent most of our time outside, which I loved. I could build and create to my heart's content. I would work on three tree houses at a time, build things out of wood, or get into other shenanigans. I remember ideas spilling out of my head at a pretty young age, but I don't remember for sure when they started coming out too fast. I remember that kids would flock around and watch me draw, build, and create as young as age five. I thought nothing of it then, but now it seems odd that I continuously created multiple things with fifteen or twenty kids watching me. I took my abilities for granted and it didn't stop.

I didn't feel different as a youngster. John liked to take things apart and put them back together. Larry could run real fast. Dan played basketball like a pro. Paul told a lot of wonderful jokes. Janet remembered everything she heard. Dana thrived on ideas, drew pictures, told stories, and sometimes struggled to find words. We were all a little different.

For me, keeping thoughts together and staying on task has always been a struggle. As a youngster, I didn't mind the fact that people couldn't keep up with my thought processing. Hell, I couldn't keep up with it either. I often forgot the point of my sentence before I finished it. I'm sure there were people who thought of me as stupid, or thought I didn't have it all together. But growing up, I noticed that kids were more accepting of a little wandering thoughts than adults. They didn't get annoyed or make heavy sighs if I shifted from topic to topic. For kids, I think it made life more interesting.

As a child, it would sometimes take me a long time to finish a thought or a sentence. Sometimes people, often adults, would get frustrated with it and start to finish my sentences for me. Now, remember, they were talking to a person with rapid thought. This kid developed more ideas in his head in a day (not always good ones, but more), than a lot of the other kids. If someone tried to finish my sentence, that meant they were finishing my thought or idea. Of course, this pissed me off. But being a passive kid, I always let it fly. When I became an adult I would sometimes speak up for myself and finish my thoughts, but not always. Therefore, I would sometimes walk away from conversations upset. Because I didn't say anything about it, nobody ever noticed the frustration.

But I do think they noticed me struggling to bring my ideas together from time to time.

When I got older, around fourteen or fifteen, I grew to six feet tall, but only weighed 140 pounds. I stayed that way for quite a while. This kind of "different" made me stand out. Sometimes I think people were so busy noticing my lanky attributes that they didn't notice some of the bipolar tendencies that I now recognize. When I was about fifteen, my father noticed a bread tie on the counter. We were sitting down to eat hamburgers and Dad decided to put the bread tie in my food when I looked away. He figured I'd take a bite and it would be funny. About twenty seconds later, I finished my hamburger and my Father wondered what happened to the bread tie. He knew I ate faster than anyone he'd ever seen, but he didn't know I would chomp down the hamburger without noticing the bread tie. Later in my life I found out that bipolar people tend to eat abnormally fast. Since my Father didn't know about bipolar, he put the bread tie in my food. Everything came out all right, by the way.

At my high school every spring, there was an extra calendar week. Since they needed to balance the semesters they held an event they called "Mini-Session," something we all looked forward to. During "Mini-Session" they offered special classes like carpentry, guitar, cooking, or anything the teachers enjoyed as a hobby that they could present for a week. Students could take those classes as enrichment to their regular routine. For one of my mini-session classes, I took Model Building. My father bought me a model car to build. Trying to contain my excitement, I took it to school. I ended up doing a less than satisfactory job on it, in my own mind. I got thumb prints on the paint and kind of hurried through it. I'd done better work on models in the past. Of course, my Dad asked me about it later so I told him the teacher wanted me to keep it at the school. I couldn't let him know I didn't meet my own expectations (or his) so I made up a story about it. I felt bad about it then and forgot about it until now, but I believe my high expectations made it difficult for me to accept substandard work. I felt a terrible amount of guilt for lying to my Dad about it, but couldn't bring myself to show him the sloppy work I'd done. Perfection and a strong work ethic were instilled into me by my family at a very young age. I carried it into just about everything I did.

When you're sixteen, a car is a car. It doesn't matter what kind it is, how many miles it has on it, or what it looks like. I bought my first car from my brother. Happy to own my first vehicle, I bought it, brought it home, and then realized it would need some attention. A fine piece of rolling stock if you ever saw one, but for me, it needed a lot of work. I sanded it, put on a new door, painted it, repainted the wheels, cleaned up the engine, cleaned the interior, recarpeted it and just about anything else I could do to make it better. I washed it almost every day and drove the hell out of it almost every night. One time, I put it up on ramps to work on it. A couple of days later, a friend came up to me and said, "What's wrong with your car? I saw it up on the ramps." I said, "Nothing." He gave me a puzzled look and walked away. It never occurred to him that I could be working on my car for the fun of it. It was part of my lifelong need to create, build, and work on something. Suddenly, I had something to work on whenever I wanted to, so I did. I could change the oil, clean the carburetor, rotate the tires, or whatever I wanted, just to keep busy. To this day, I've made it a point to have as many cars in my life as possible. I found therapy and I didn't even know it.

I went away to college at the age of nineteen and every month or two I would return home to visit. Quite often on my visits home I would take rides up the shore of Lake Michigan with a pint of whiskey in my pocket or a joint in my hand and stop to look at the lake. I would sometimes go for walks on the beach or just sit and look at the water, emptying the whiskey bottle before making my way to my family home. I never thought about it until now, but taking these little "side trips" might be appropriate for someone who long since left the area, but for a nineteen-year-old who visited every other month or so, it might have been a little out of the norm. This down time may have been a way for the "busy kid" to unwind a little before going home. It also might have been a subconscious way for me to bring down some of the mania I never even knew existed.

When it came to the opposite sex, I never seemed to have a shortage of girlfriends. Being tall and lanky, I didn't have the makings of a "ladies man" in any way, but I dated a lot in spite of my attributes. I may have intimidated some of the women I dated. I didn't play the field, so to speak, as I tended to date one girl at a time. But because of my high energy level, I believe I might have smothered them a little. Some women like being smothered and some don't, but what I see now that I know a little bit about bipolar disorder is that I may have been a little overbearing. When people have manic episodes, they sometimes become promiscuous or try to dominate relationships. Having lived with a high level of mania in my life thus far, that may have been the case.

Then there was Kris. At about eighteen, I developed a crush on a girl named Kris. A bunch of us worked in the dining room at a nearby hotel. She waited tables and I bussed them. As anyone can imagine, I flew around the dining room at full speed. I must've been paying too much attention to Kris, for another worker started singing, "Speedy Gonzales, leave that Kris alone!" He sang it as if singing it to the world but I knew he aimed it at me. He then looked at Kris and said, "What do you think of that, Kris?" It seemed like a directive for me to pay less attention to Kris and it did hurt. But later as I thought about it, I realized other people were noticing the mania. Of course, since I'd known the other worker for years, I wondered why he didn't just tell me Kris didn't care for my extra attention. Perhaps, because we were such young men, he avoided the confrontation. But now as I've gotten older, I realize people were noticing my mania at a time when I didn't.

For thirty years, no one came right out and mentioned it. No one noticed mood swings. They saw no ups and downs or anger. They didn't notice any depression or long periods of sadness. The reason is, it just didn't happen. With a typical bipolar person, there are cycles. Not the kind you drive, but the kind you ride with your mind. There are ups and downs that are difficult, if not impossible to control. Someone who is bipolar can go and go for days, but sooner or later they're going to crash. When they're up, people flock around them. Many people experiencing manic episodes are great to be around. They're funny as hell and have a million ideas about what to do next. But when they're down, it's not as great. I didn't know about that yet. I would later learn of the darkness, loneliness, and cold. So far for me, I only knew one direction. Up.

5

OBSESS MUCH?

I *got up early on a Monday morning and ran to*
the Music Building at the university I attended
to find a practice room and begin the day. The custodian
turned the key in the lock and I burst in and ran up the
stairs to find the practice room with my favorite piano in it.
Soon after I began practicing all of the music I needed for
my end-of-the-year festivities, the rest of the building came
to life. I could hear xylophones, pianos, horns, and voices
echoing throughout the halls. What a wonderful place to be
and what a wonderful time in my life! I practiced almost
with abandon, trying to fit everything in before my first
class. I moved frantically through choral pieces, arias, vocal
jazz charts, and even barbershop quartet songs. When I
finished, I pushed the door open like a starting gate and
headed on my way.

Once in class, I couldn't concentrate, much like other days,
but this time my mind wandered more than usual. I was in the
process of preparing for a musical performance that would

soon be upon me, and could think of little else. Would my music be memorized in time? Would I have solos, quartets, and other ensembles ready to perform at the level they needed to be? With a million thoughts and ideas in my mind, I couldn't focus on German like I should. My teacher asked, "Sind sie in Ordnung?" I replied "Mein regen schirm ist kaputt!" She asked me if I was okay and "My umbrella is broken" was the only thing I remembered from an entire semester of German. But soon, German class came to an end and I raced across campus to my first rehearsal of the day.

I looked forward to the biggest concert of the year. There were six ensembles performing in the concert and I partici-pated in five of them. The Madrigal Singers, a Vocal Jazz Ensemble, the Men's Glee Club, a Barbershop Quartet, and the Concert Choir were all important parts of my life. When the Men's Glee Club performed, I trembled with excitement because I would perform my first major solo on the main audi-torium stage. I guess I forgot that I would be performing in a Barbershop Quartet the very next act. I'd already been on the stage in three other ensembles. I went backstage, changed my shirt, ran behind the set and walked back onto the stage to meet the rest of the quartet. The audience must have been getting used to seeing my face. As I stepped on the stage to perform, they broke into laughter. We accepted it and started our first song.

What a good life so far. I could work, play, and create just about all of the time without writer's blocks or lulls that seemed to get in other people's way. I partied without knowing about hangovers. I balanced family, friends and work into it all. At twenty-two years old I was running myself ragged and didn't even know it. Knee-deep in music school, I worked my tail off trying to graduate, partied like crazy with friends and ate if I remembered to. I only slept when necessary. I enjoyed every minute of it. I worked at a bar where I could run at full speed and drink after work with coworkers. I lived in a house full of guys who enjoyed my zany antics. I soon moved into a smaller apartment with just one roommate for my senior year and then life started to get interesting.

I dated a girl I'd met in the music department at school, but for some reason, there were a lot of other women in my life. They weren't girlfriends. They were just women who were interested in me. I didn't often get this kind of attention from women. A girl in the apartment below me, a longtime friend, my "girlfriend," and another girl from the music department were all hovering around my romantic scene. It overwhelmed me. Then it happened. I met the woman whom I would spend the rest of my life with. I knew it for sure. I didn't get down on one knee and propose right then and there, but I knew I met the girl I'd be with forever and broke up with my girlfriend so I could date her. This important event changed my life forever.

After I met this girl, I shifted into overdrive. We spent all of our time together when we weren't in school. We would run home between classes to spend time together and be with each other every night. Everyone and everything else seemed to be put on hold. I'd never been this overcome by someone before. We got married within a year and we both graduated from college. Soon after that we started our family. We did everything for each other and our new little family. But I needed to think about my professional life again.

At the time, I tended bar for a living and because of my elevated mood, I ran around the bar like a wild man. The owners of the restaurant stayed out of my way and let me run the bar on my own. My system worked well and I was a tireless worker. But my wife and I were both trained teachers, so as soon as we could we moved to the Detroit area for a year, then settled in a small town south of Grand Rapids where we lived for five years watching our family grow from one child to three. As I was quite productive, this may have been the best time in my life.

My twenty-seventh year came and thoughts and ideas still oozed out of me. Even though I had grown older I still bubbled with ideas and energy. We moved into our first home, and it needed work. It would be easier to say it didn't need a roof or windows. But I didn't look at it as a home improvement project. I saw it as a big science project. Since money didn't grow on trees, the home got rebuilt out of a lot of recycled material. The doghouse looked good compared to the house. But soon there were Dutch doors, custom countertops, and handmade surprises all over the place. My wife worked with me every day to rebuild it. At night I would continue to work and the neighbors would put up with the noise from my hammers and saws. They could count on something happening at our house 24/7.

When I first began teaching, I would stay awake at night building toys for the kids, writing music, working on the house, and thinking of ways to make my school lessons more interesting. My father gave me a set of old "Popular Mechanics" books with ideas and plans for building storage units, heaters, toys, tools, stereos, and just about anything else I could think of. Now remember, I could think of a lot, and the set contained about ten books, so closet organizers, work benches, pulley systems, and bird houses were everywhere. My family loved it. I built and created frantically. Good humor, creativity, and productivity poured out of me. At work, the principal called me the "Pied Piper." I taught music for grades one through seven and worked with kids on singing and performing. We did all-school performances that were fun and entertaining. The kids came to performances in costume and so did I. If we performed an oldies show, Elvis Presley made an appearance. If we performed a country music show, there were 400 cowboy hats. Each performance was packed to the gills, with nowhere to park, but even though the shows were talked about for weeks after they happened, I needed more.

An opportunity for a new job came up that would take us to a beautiful spot on the west side of the state. It would take us closer to Lake Michigan, give me a chance to work with a K – 12 Program, and settle us in a small community, which would be a great place to raise our family. I interviewed for it and received an offer, so we went. We packed up our lives and moved again.

On my first day, a scant thirteen kids were in the high school choir. I'd seen "fixer uppers" before, so I knew what to do, but I did have some work ahead of me. The band program at the school flourished with ninety students, but twenty years had gone by with no choir program until I showed up. I started fresh and the first year went well because the few kids I taught were dedicated to helping me build a program. I always felt sorry for them because I knew there were great opportunities to come after they were gone, but they were the ones who laid the foundation.

I loved my new job. Because of the absence of a choral program in this town, or any town in the county, in so many years, everything we did went over very well. Being the new kid on the block and a big fish in a small pond, I loved every minute of it. At this point, I worked around the clock. Starting a new program meant spending a lot of time at work. My energy level soared, but I slighted my family and didn't realize it.

As the number of students in the choirs grew, so did the program. The kids went on tours, did a catered dinner revue, and much more. Soon, the Shelby High School Concert Choir grew to more than eighty students. We did shows with impressive special effects, interesting props, and talented soloists. But here's the thing - if I did a show, I might have a thousand ideas I wanted to incorporate into it. But because of budget and facility restrictions, among other issues, I often pulled off only about three hundred of those ideas. While that seems awesome, when you're an overachiever, it's sometimes difficult to accept a project with a third of your ideas in it. I would have people come up to me after a show and praise the hell out of it, after which I would thank them, but in my head I thought, "you should've seen what I pictured in my mind."

It shames me to say it, but I became obsessed with my work. I shut out my family and friends. I didn't make room for a social life, a home life, or personal interests. For a while, for a very long while, I worked constantly. I'm sure my family grew tired of it. I see now that I didn't deserve my wife's patience. Looking back, I remember manic times when I would cross the line in social settings. I might drink too much and jump off the roof, or tell jokes and stories that offended people. I wasn't angry often, but it happened on occasion. I would sometimes swear for no apparent reason or throw things. As a teacher, especially in my first few years, I might give the students a tongue lashing they didn't deserve. Debbie would often find the need to set me straight. These outbreaks caused enough friction in our marriage to the point where we almost lost it. Fortunately, I was able to get the outbreaks under control with medication and we were able to get through the hard times.

When my own children were old enough to participate in my music classes, it became easier, because at least then they were included in my life and my projects. I would get up early so I could get to work and stay late to help students with their music. I'd often work nights and weekends on staging. I even started to dream of my job on a regular basis. I would often wake up in the night thinking about work and start creating. I arranged much of the music we performed myself with definite ideas about what the kids should perform and how they performed it.

At this time in my life, I seldom did any building or creating at home. Most of my creative energy went to my job. I still cleaned and painted and did some things around the house, but there were no more inventions. There were no more handmade closet organizers with hidden shoe racks or under-the-bed Barbie cases on wheels with dividers for dolls and clothes. I'm not sure, but I think I slowed down and didn't realize it. I think that at around age thirty-two, depression started to appear, but instead of becoming flat out "depressed," I adapted by channeling all of my energy into one place. I'd basically bubbled over with mania up until this point, but since I'd never cycled, no one diagnosed me with anything. That said, if you run an engine at full speed long enough, it's going to run out of gas.

But I didn't run out of gas. Not yet, at least. I kept teaching and performing. I kept pushing myself and my students as hard and far as I could. At this point, I loved being on the stage with young people and they responded very well. I'd never been sick a day in my life so I just kept pushing. I kept on creating, working, and running myself into the ground. I didn't know I ran myself into the ground. In my opinion, I just worked the way everyone else did. Since I'd run at full throttle all my life, working this way seemed normal to me. But soon would come the setback, the moment when just a regular day with my son cuddled on my lap turned full circle for me. In the blink of an eye my life changed forever.

6

IF IT LOOKS LIKE A SEIZURE...

hy was he sitting at the table eating a hamburger all alone? With his head down, he looked like a whipped pup. I went to the bar and ordered a stiff drink. "Give me my usual iced tea, no lemon" I said. I snapped up my drink and went to sit across the table from Lyle, a student of mine, who was picking away at his hamburger.

"What's the trouble?" I asked him. When you live in a small town and you've taught as many years as I, you know just about everyone. I'd known him for several years and felt comfortable talking to him. Something seemed wrong.

He looked over his glasses and said, "I'm gonna be a father." I nodded to him and just let him talk. He continued, "I've made a lot of mistakes in my life, but this is the biggest one ever!"

I looked at him, gave him just a slight smile and asked, "Are you married?"

He replied, "No, and I don't know if I want to be. This is just a girlfriend of mine and something that randomly happened. It's the biggest mistake I ever made."

I sipped my iced tea for a few moments and then I started talking to him like a dad. "You know, Lyle, I've made a few mistakes in my own life. But out of all the things I've done, I have three things I am the most proud of. I have three things I wouldn't trade for anything in the world. I wouldn't trade them for a million dollars. Those three things are Michael, Erin, and David." He knew all of my kids and he looked up and smiled. I continued, saying, "Even though this might not be the best time for you, I believe when you hold your child for the first time, you won't think he or she is a mistake. Now, whether or not things will work out with this young lady, I can't tell you. But this child needs to go through life knowing he has a father who loves him. One day, when you're on the couch with that newborn child on your chest snuggling into you, you'll feel nothing but love. All I'm saying is give this some time and I think you'll find it's the BEST mistake you ever made." I patted him on the back and walked away.

A couple of years later I saw Lyle and he came up to me with a wallet full of pictures of his daughter. He said, "You were right, Mr. Wall. She's the best thing that ever happened to me. I have no regrets." Those words were music to my ears, and I knew, because of my relationship with my own children, that all he needed to do was hold her for the first time.

I worked around the clock and didn't always come up for air like I should have. But being a good Dad still came easy to me. I always took great pride in my three children and I'm proud to say I've been a part of who they've become. My youngest, David, sat on my lap listening to a story when my first "episode" or "seizure" came. I remember some of it, but became very confused when it ended. I got a real bad metallic taste in my mouth and then a strong head rush happened. I don't know how much time passed. Several seconds would go by and then I would wake up confused and ask questions that didn't make sense. I couldn't remember where I was, what day it was, if I worked, if I needed to make dinner, etc. The questions I would ask were often random and unrelated. Some time went by before this happened again. As time went by it began happening more frequently. One day it happened in the classroom. I went home from work early and called my doctor. While on the phone with the receptionist she said, "Can you come in right now?" I agreed, and she said, "You just called a minute ago and made an appointment. Don't you remember?" I said, "No." She then said, "I think it's important for you to come in right now." So I went.

My doctor ordered an MRI of my brain and referred me to a neurologist. The neurologist found scar tissue on my brain which may have been from an old stroke and gave me seizure medication. I'm not sure about this, but I always thought this neurologist just needed a new set of golf clubs. I never felt as though he tried very hard to diagnose anything. The episode didn't seem like any seizure I'd heard of. But, the neurologist told me to take Dilantin (phenytoin), so I did. The "seizures" went away for a while. I didn't like that they called this "episode" a "seizure" because I didn't have convulsions. But because of my practical personality, I took my Dilantin like a good boy, and ignored the fact that I didn't think they were seizures. I went on with my life.

I continued to work but found I didn't have the same familiar spark that I used to have. In 1998, while at work one day, I just didn't feel right. I went to the vending machine to get a soda and some candy because I felt as though a little caffeine or sugar may pick me up. A little later, I got that same familiar head rush, only more intense than in the past. I asked my student aid to go get the principal. I told him that I couldn't see the kids. I got double vision and couldn't concentrate. I began to slur my speech and I didn't make much sense. The school counselor drove me to the doctor. He and his staff were all over me the minute I got in the door. Soon my wife came and my doctor drove us in our car, ninety miles an hour, talking on the Bat Phone all the way to the nearest large city, and put me in the hospital. It appeared to be a stroke and he wanted to try to reverse it. I have a good relationship with my doctor, so all the way there I told him dirty jokes with a slow speaking voice. He didn't appreciate it or understand it, but it kept me busy so he ignored me and kept driving.

Afterwards, we found it to be a TIA (Transient Ischemic Attack) or mini-stroke. I spent the night in the hospital and a physical therapist came to check me over, as well as a speech therapist. My speech had become delayed the day before so they needed someone to come in and make sure I could speak in complete sentences. After a long day and a very sleepless night, my wife and I needed to make some decisions. We decided to let my regular doctor take complete control of all my medical needs and handle all of my medication himself. He felt a medication change would help.

Changing medication is a bitch. In my vast experience, medications can't simply be changed just like that. If it's a mood altering medication, one has to start with a small dose of it, then give a blood sample to see how much is in the bloodstream. Then the doctor administers a little more or less and the process is repeated until the medication is just right. When one changes medications, they have to go off of one gradually and then go on the new medication gradually, as well. If the patient happens to be a pain in the ass when they're not on the medication, then everyone has to deal with them during the transition. If a seizure disorder is part of the equation then the patient is at risk of having a seizure during this time. It's hell for everyone.

My doctor prescribed Elavil (amitriptyline) next. Most often used as an antidepressant, Elavil would likely eliminate stress as a way to curb the "seizures." I had not been diagnosed with bipolar disorder at this point, so I used Elavil only to prevent the "seizures." I went for quite a while without having a seizure while taking this drug, and I continued working without any problem. Also, when I first started taking this medication I slept a little better. This overjoyed me because I never slept much. But the sleep benefit that came from Elavil soon wore off and I returned to my regular pattern once again. It's worth noting that I wrote a significant percentage of this book in the middle of the night.

When my doctor prescribed Elavil I think he stumbled onto something important. He used a drug to treat me for "seizures" that is often used as an antidepressant. What a great piece of "candy" to give to an undiagnosed bipolar man. When I look back over more than twenty years, I believe this is what kept me from getting into a hell of a lot of trouble at a very difficult time in my life. Although I hadn't been depressed before, it had become difficult to stay positive and create. After I took Elavil for a while, my ability to create seemed to revive. I started to have energy again and began to restore my "think tank." Thank God! Being Dana meant having lots of ideas in my head. Those ideas were part of the reason for my success as a teacher.

The seizures were now under control and I still wanted to create quality performances at work. I continued to build unnecessary things. I still labeled everything from the radio antenna to the water fountain. My student aids would help me file music, because at that time, I couldn't keep it filed neatly enough or often enough.

We did a choral music revue in the spring, which encompassed around fifty songs. A lot of groups would have the students stand and sing with their folders in their hands. But my choir didn't. My choir learned them all from memory and sang and danced to every beat. We incorporated twenty solos into each show and almost every soloist wore a costume. Props and sets were also very important to me. For instance, if we performed a disco revue, I needed to build a lighted disco floor for the soloists to dance on. But it also needed to be tilted so the audience could see it. When we did a country music revue, I built a giant barn for the background of the finale with students jumping out of the hayloft. The shows were big, loud, and fun. At this point, things were running smoothly once again.

"Normality" seemed to be falling back into place...for me. I got up in the morning at a decent time. I went to work early, stayed late, and worked as hard as I could. Just like before, I would obsess over my job. I made very little time for my family, very little time for myself, and very little time for anything or anyone else. I didn't mind being away from home so often. It didn't bother anyone. Right? WRONG! I found out some time later that it ticked my wife off a lot when I didn't make enough time for her or the kids. Since we were both teachers, we traveled a lot in the summer, but it didn't make up for time lost day-to-day. I often spent too much time centered on work. When I became ill with the so-called seizure disorder, I couldn't wait to get one thing over with so I could find something else to get busy with. Finding things to do kept my mind off of my illness and gave me a sense of focus. I loved getting ready for performances and losing myself in the excitement of the preparation. That's what I did.

7

HOW LOW CAN YOU GO?

he "Snooze Button" is the last little breath of freedom before we start our day. It is the one last bit of control we have before starting a busy cycle. We can just lean over, give it a slap, and drift off for ten more minutes before taking on all of the trials and tribulations involved in the regular chaos of life. What is the proper amount of times to hit a "snooze" button? Should it be one or two? Six or seven seemed to be a more appropriate number. But Saturday came. Don't you want to get up and enjoy your day off? Don't you want to leave the "snooze" button out of it, jump to your feet, and breathe the fresh morning air? I can breathe just fine here on my mattress, thank you very much.

And lay on the mattress I did. Around noon, I would curl out of my "cocoon" and stagger to my feet to find something to eat before making my way to the television set. Some people have a quick trigger finger and are an excellent shot with a pistol or rifle. With a quick trigger THUMB I became a sharpshooter with the remote control. I could flip from channel to channel with lightning speed or adjust the volume on a dime. I could run that television like a marksman and even knew how to gauge commercials for length, giving me just enough time for a break to the kitchen or an occasional jog to the bathroom. Fred Flintstone, Fred Rogers, and Fred Astaire became close friends of mine.

Later in the day I might make my way to the computer where I'd stare at the screen for a while. The glow would feel warm against my skin and the images on the screen would occupy my time for hours on end. I would surf from place to place and enjoy the freedom and confinement it gave me. After a while, I might slither back to the couch, find the remote control that I loved so well and start the process all over again. What an odd place for a hyperactive person to spend his Saturday. Mania seemed like a distant memory. I got nothing done, and I just didn't care.

Mania is often defined as an abnormally elevated mood, arousal, or energy level, and most of the time my personality leaned in this direction. For people who are manic, the upside is they feel great! If they're a creative person, they often have ideas exploding out of their heads. If they're athletic, they can run like hell. Manic people are often fun to be around, except not all of them are happy. Sometimes an elevated mood can be irritable. The mood is elevated, but it comes out as anger. That wasn't the case with me. I could get along with anyone and had a high level of productivity. Or so I thought.

I do want to take a look at this so-called productivity. If a man is awake at three o'clock in the morning alphabetizing his videotapes and baking cookies because he can't sleep, it doesn't mean he's being productive. I thought it did, but I've come to realize differently. Putting a sign on the trash can that says "Don't forget to feed the waste basket" and another one on the stapler saying "Punch Me," is not a valuable use of time. But a full-grown "busy" kid may sometimes let those kinds of things take priority over others. And for me, the "busy" light just didn't burn out, until now.

At the age of about thirty-five, I found it became more difficult for me to concentrate than in the past. Sometimes, if someone asked me a question, I would appear to stare right through them while I thought of my answer. I would space out for a moment while I considered their question, go into a world of my own, and then come back and answer it. Those delays weren't long, and my brain didn't shut down. I just needed more concentration time than I used to. At work, I still thought of myself as an "Idea Factory." We were creating wonderful shows and beautiful music. But I would often drift off and didn't know why. In a social setting, if my wife and I were having dinner with another couple, I may lose concentration and drift out of the conversation. She would give my leg a squeeze under the table to get me back on task. It happened more than I wanted to admit. It pissed me off when she nudged me or squeezed me. It didn't bother me so much that she did it, but that it needed to be done.

At home, I would require more alone time than I ever needed before. I set up a massive fifty-gallon fish tank and would just sit and look at the fish for hours. If you go to an aquarium, you look at one tank for five minutes or so then move along to another one. I gazed at the same damned tank of fish in my basement for hours on end, even days. Sometimes I would listen to the gurgle of the water and just gaze right on past the glass. Watching the fish tank became a regular part of my routine and I spent a lot of time alone there. For someone never able to sit still for five straight minutes before in his life, things were changing. I often got bored with the fish tank and found other things to occupy my time.

When I wasn't staring at the fish tank, I might sit out on the front porch with a cocktail in my hand. I drank quite a bit in college, but not like this. I would drink whiskey and sit on the front porch watching the road on a regular basis. I had a decanter full on the counter and a cupboard full of it but still had to replenish it often. Because some of my neighbors were students, I put my whiskey in a big colored tumbler to disguise it. I started to hide my liquor and might have been developing a problem. But I kept doing it. I would often sit on the tailgate of my pickup truck and watch the stars as well. When there were no stars, I just gazed up at the sky. My wife bought me a telescope to stargaze with. She thought it would give me some direction instead of just sitting in the back of the truck. But stars and planets don't move very fast, so I would get one into view and back onto the tailgate I'd climb, whiskey in hand. For a "busy" kid, sitting on the porch alone or in the back of my truck watching the stars and drinking whiskey kind of broke the pattern.

But that's what I did, for weeks and months at a time. When I took those breaks and went into a world of my own, I found it to be very dark. I frequently wondered whether the world would be a better place without me in it. The thoughts in my head and the places I went in my mind were gut wrenching and horrible. During bouts with depression, I often thought of myself as useless. I didn't talk about it then and don't talk about it now because the thoughts I had were personal and scary. Having never been depressed a day in my life, I would now slip into cold, dark places for days and weeks at a time. I didn't realize I was beginning to cycle.

A bipolar cycle is the period of time when a person goes between mania and depression. The question that comes up quite often is how long it takes for a person to run a full cycle. The answer to that question is quite simple: "I DON'T KNOW!" The length of a bipolar cycle is undetermined and varies from person to person. It even varies from cycle to cycle. Some people have mixed bipolar symptoms, which means they can be both manic and depressed at the same time. But people with mixed bipolar symptoms don't always cycle in this way. That's why bipolar disorder is so hard to diagnose and treat. In my experience, knowing how often or how long a bipolar person will cycle is very hard to determine. When my wife, Debbie, and I talk about my early stages of depression, she says she didn't notice any problems. I think she concerned herself more with the amount of alcohol I drank and credited my behavior to that.

At this point, I started to cycle drastically but wasn't always aware, or didn't admit it was happening. I believe I drank whiskey as a form of self medication for the depression I didn't know existed. I didn't have any other excuse for drinking it. This theory makes pretty good sense, since many undiagnosed bipolar people self medicate. They aren't always aware of it, but tobacco and alcohol, along with other drugs, often take the edge off of a pretty spicy personality brought on by bipolar. So I continued on this way for some time, and I got rather good at it.

But one day, right after the spring concert, my health changed. I went into work in very low gear. My skin radiated a yellow hue and I felt worn out. I'd just arrived and the principal told me to go to the doctor. He took one look at me and knew. My doctor discovered my thyroid level to be low. My thyroid gland stopped working. This meant I would have to go on a very strong dose of Synthroid (levothyroxine) to replace the thyroid that was no longer producing. When on such a strong dose of Synthroid, in addition to my other medications, I wasn't supposed to drink alcohol, so I didn't. It was difficult for me, but I immediately stopped drinking.

It took me a while to get my thyroid level adjusted, but I soon got my energy level back on track and went back to work. I still did my job. For some reason or another, I could get up and go. I could still create great shows and pick good music. Somehow, ideas continued to flow and I came up with one of my biggest ones. I wasn't sure the timing was right, but I wanted to do it anyway.

Armed with all the tools I needed to create something special, I damned well set out to do it. When I got something in my head, no one could change my mind. I often became obsessed with these creations and my family would just stand by and watch. I thought and talked about little else for weeks at a time. Since this project would last about a year, my wife and kids were going to be drastically affected. I wrapped myself up in the project and never noticed. I just kept on moving.

8

OUT OF GAS!

I would soon start thinking about my biggest project of the year. We would present our dinner choral revue, a catered event performed over two nights that soon became the highlight of the year. We served 250 people each night. We offered a wonderful prime rib dinner and the students in the choir waited tables. With the event being somewhat formal and sophisticated, our small town looked forward to it. I produced sixteen of these revues over the years while working in the small western Michigan town of Shelby. After dinner, the audience would move into the auditorium where the choir would present a revue of non-stop musical medleys lasting from forty-five minutes to an hour. Every year we did a different theme and the students would dress, sing, and dance accordingly. This year would be no exception.

I wanted to do a country music revue. Except there

wasn't one. No company ever arranged a revue of this kind. I searched everywhere. I even thought about using individual songs and linking them together but found out there wasn't much country music available for choirs.

I decided I wanted to do one anyway and set out to write the whole thing myself. There are people who do this for a living, so it's not a big deal, and I'd composed many pieces in college and felt I should be able to pull it off. I purchased a program for the computer so I could both write the show and play the accompaniment back. It would play drums, banjo, horns, guitars, bass, piano, and more. But since I still needed to do my job, writing the show might have been an unrealistic goal. After all, the people who did such work for a living only had ONE JOB! I see that now, but back then I couldn't see the flaw. My family felt that it was out of my grasp but didn't say anything.

With a lot to learn, the choir would start working on music and choreography just after the Christmas concert and present the show in mid March. This meant I needed to have the music ready by about December 10. Well, let me dial back a little and see how that all played out. I started working on the music at the beginning of the summer and things were going a little slow. I just couldn't create. I'd chosen many of the songs I wanted to include in the revue and then outlined them into sections or medleys. From there, I would write them into three or four vocal parts and arrange the accompaniment. November rolled around and the music still needed an immense amount of work. We were working on producing the Christmas concert by now and I didn't have time to work on the country show.

After the Christmas concert, I crashed. My mind went empty and I broke down. I became exhausted and couldn't go forward or backward. I'm not sure what happened, but my mind became empty. The idea of finishing the music overwhelmed me. I'd barely even started arranging and I would soon need to teach it. Completely wiped out, I only had one week of school left before Christmas break. I didn't know what else to do, so I went to the superintendent and asked for a week off. I explained that I simply couldn't move forward. For some reason, he understood. He sensed I needed time to get myself together, so I stayed home and worked on the music, but mania comes at unexpected times and works in mysterious ways, so the country show wasn't the only thing on my mind.

"Announcing: The 12th Annual Festival of the Trees! The Friends of the Library will be accepting donations from anyone who would like to decorate and donate a tree. All trees will be auctioned off and the money will be donated for the good of the Village Library."

What a fantastic idea! I began creating a music themed tree, decorated with hand-carved miniature electric guitars and little records all made of wood. I worked for about a month, cutting out guitars, sanding them, staining them, and painting them. They were all different and stained or painted to look like a brand name guitar. Little wooden discs were hung on the tree to look like records, accompanied by garland made of music notes and symbols.

As I thought about it, I wanted an artificial pre-lit tree so the new owner could enjoy it for years to come. A star or an angel did not seem like an appropriate tree top for a rock-and-roll themed tree, so a wooden cut-out of a treble clef painted with silver and glitter sat atop this glorious creation. As I looked at the nearly complete Christmas tree, I thought putting gift boxes at the bottom would provide a nice place to store the instruments and records when the tree wasn't in use. Better yet, boxes which looked like AMPLIFIERS would be even better. I wrapped the boxes in black paper with rubber handles riveted to the top and grills pasted to the side. It was wonderful...but still not complete. I needed a tree skirt to finish the ensemble, so I went to several fabric stores looking for just the right music themed fabric to complete the job. After a lot of searching, I found a fabric covered in black and white notes and symbols that would look beautiful underneath the tree. Not being a seamstress, it took a while to create the tree skirt, but once done, it lay underneath the tiny tree, pulling all of the elements together. Finally, the time had come to take the tree to the "Festival of Trees" and unveil it.

Not being one with a lot of spare time, it seems odd that I wanted to create the tree in the first place. But something lit a fire under me and told me I should do it, I should spend every waking hour working on a Christmas tree that would be auctioned off for just a little less than what I put into it. Something told me to do this and all of my other important tasks would be put on hold. That something was mania!

During the week I spent at home, I somehow slipped into overdrive. I got a burst of energy and began doing anything and everything. I started labeling things that didn't need to be labeled. I built random things and worked on unrelated projects. It's clear now that a manic cycle wound me up tight. I found things to do besides the task I'd stayed home to do. I worked on the show too, but my behavior became a little random and unpredictable, even for me. According to my family, I spoke very fast, skipping from topic to topic and went with very little sleep. I moved around quickly, almost frantically, but didn't accomplish much. I did a lot of unnecessary things. I cooked and baked at two o'clock in the morning and built things I didn't need out in the garage night and day.

I enjoyed writing the show, though. I spent a lot of time on it and it became challenging and fun. I set up three keyboard voices in the computer so I could hear what the choir would sound like when they sang the music and what the other instruments would play, as well. Once in a while students would stop by to see how things were going and I would play it for them. They were amazed how so much sound could come out of the computer. Since I'd never arranged anything of this magnitude, I shared their amazement. The show consisted of five different medleys. They were all different country music themes. One might be "Songs of Love", another might be "Songs of Old", and so on. Once completed, more than fifty songs were represented in the revue.

While at home, I began building the barn. The barn would be the backdrop for the finale of the show. I would build a big platform and put the barn up there. Then students could dance in it, sing solos, and make announcements. I'm not sure how I got the barn to the school after I got it built. I'm guessing I took it there in a couple of pieces in the back of my truck. The show took place in March of 2002, so it's a little hard for me to remember the details. It's important for me to remember the dates, though. During this year in particular, many things started to unravel. I came to a complete stand-still in December of 2001. I'd never been in such a state of emotional and physical exhaustion before.

I remember talking to my wife, Debbie, about it and I cried. That's a big deal, because I never cried much. Debbie always said I had a high tolerance for pain. If I got a cold or the flu or something, I would be the biggest baby in the world, but if I cut off one of my fingertips, I might say, "Well, I've got nine more."

At this point, I came to a halt, my mind filled with overwhelming thoughts. I felt as though I'd lost. I set out to create a piece of music and wasn't able to do it. Luckily, my boss understood and gave me the time I needed to go into lockup and work on it. He didn't ask me any questions about my health or my personal life. He just trusted me and let me go. I'm glad he didn't ask me anything, because I didn't have any answers. I didn't know why I couldn't create during the summer. I just couldn't. For some reason, ideas were not coming out as easily as they had in the past and I didn't have the energy I used to. I wanted to do all of the work and outlined it in my mind, but when I sat down to work on it, nothing came out. By Christmastime, I felt backed against a wall and needed to be alone.

I just needed to sit around in my bathrobe and write music without any interruptions. I needed to focus all of my energy and concentration on something I'd neglected for a long time. Sometimes it would flow from my fingertips like fine wine and other times it moved a little more like molasses. But I kept writing, erasing, cutting, pasting, and swearing, until I completed the show. I became very manic and difficult to get along with during this time. I'm sure if you talked with my family about it, they'd recall the situation in a different way. They might describe my temperament and mood swings in ways other than I recall. When I listen to them tell what happened, I understand that my mania and mood swings were severe, though I got more done in that week off than I'd done in six-and-a-half months. I continued to work into Christmas break and when I got back to school in January, I taught the music and the students were ready to work on the choreography.

Proud of my accomplishment, I still felt some sort of a void inside of me. Something made it difficult for me to create music during the summer. Something made me so frustrated that I couldn't move forward. This feeling seemed new to me. Focusing and creating became diffi-cult. When depression started to appear, I didn't admit it or acknowledge it, but now I was face to face with mental exhaustion. I went to see my regular doctor again to see what he thought.

It didn't take long to get an appointment. Because of the manic state I'd been in, they wanted to see me right away. Immediately, they sent me to the lab and took a lot of blood. They found the levels of my medications to be normal, but I didn't feel normal at all. When I saw my doctor I raised my voice a little and said, "Doc, I'm a mess! I can't think! I can't create!" I didn't have any energy or feel like doing anything! The medication seemed to be controlling the so-called seizures, but I suffered from complete exhaustion. "What the hell?" My doctor just looked at me and said, "I don't think the problem is something I can fix. I think you need to see our counselor and see if she can figure it out. From there, maybe a psychiatrist."

I didn't want to hear this at all! I didn't kick and scream because I'd seen a counselor before, but I hoped she could just write me a prescription and send me on my way. Isn't that what we all want when we go to the doctor? Just give me a handful of little purple pills and I'll be better in a week. But it didn't turn out that way.

I dragged my feet on the way out of the doctor's office and made an appointment to see a counselor. As luck would have it, she could see me right away. That didn't give me much time to kick up a fuss. I had a couple of days to be pissed off about it and then would have to go in and spill my guts to someone I didn't even know. When someone started digging around inside of my head, I became nervous about what they might find. At almost 40 years old, a lot of things were trapped in my mind. Up until now, I'd felt pretty "normal." I didn't want to go to a "shrink." What would we talk about? I didn't look forward to this at all.

9

YOU SAY YOUR WHAT HURTS?

*A*bout halfway into the fourteenth year of my life, I
sat in a study hall gazing out the window, which
*overlooked beautiful Portage Lake. I watched the boats drift by
thinking about how wonderful it would be to have a boat of
my own. Many times I thought about that, but on this particular day I decided to do something about it. I started drawing
out plans for a one-person hydroplane, thinking I could
build one.*

*Later in the day, I approached my friend, Frank, and he
liked the idea. He didn't think I knew much about building
boats but agreed to help, so we started off like two crazed scientists. Frank's family owned a cottage with a shed down by the
water and my parents would seldom come to see what we were
doing. We set out to build our watercraft.*

*We worked from March until the end of May, cutting,
sanding, drilling, nailing, and even fiberglassing, until we
completed our masterpiece. We planned to mount a small
fishing motor on the back of it. Finally, the time came to take it*

out of the shed and set it in the water for the first time. The big moment had arrived!

With all of the careful calculation we did to build our boat, it seems one of us would have noticed the service door in the shed would not be big enough to accommodate the tiny craft. Taking the boat apart seemed unrealistic so we began disassembling the door and the wall of the shed with care. We needed to be sure we could get it back together and we also wanted to be sure Frank's parents wouldn't be able to tell that we took it apart in the first place. With a lot of careful strategy, we got the wall apart, removed the boat, and put the building back together without much damage.

Sometimes, before you can get on with the good things in life, you need to open things up and see what's inside. Frank and I learned this lesson the hard way. But before long, we were taking turns out on the water in our new power boat. Through life I often look back on this lesson and remember not how stupid we were to build a boat in a building that we couldn't get it out of, but the process we went through to realize a dream.

I went to counseling looking for answers, but I didn't expect to get them. I expected to be there for weeks or months before anything happened. I took voice lessons for seven semesters before I got any results. I felt counseling would be similar. I figured I'd talk and she'd say "mm hmm, mm hmm." Then I'd come back in a week and we'd start the whole process all over again. When I got there, the therapist greeted me with a handshake, then she sat down with a pad of paper and wrote down a lot of what I said. She told me she wouldn't do that every time, but during the first session she wanted to remember my background information. She found out a lot about me.

I told her everything. I told her all about my family, my brother and two sisters. I told her about my adopted brother and the challenges of raising him. I told her about my sister's life with multiple sclerosis. I even told her about my brother's suicide. I find it odd, but the "episodes" or "seizures" started soon after his death. I developed bouts with depression at that time, as well.

My counselor found this to be very interesting. I also talked about my professional life. I told her what I did for a living and what my job responsibilities were. All of my job responsibilities were self assigned. I developed the program myself, and did things I felt were important for the students to learn. Very little of what I did was required. I told her how many concerts we did in a year. I told her how many trips we took, how much music I required the students to learn, and just about every other aspect of my job. In the middle of it all, I noticed that her eyes were open pretty wide, along with her mouth. There were eighty-five students in both my middle and high school choirs. I taught a guitar class with at least twenty-five students in it. I directed a select show choir that performed all over the county and beyond. We were working on the country music revue I wrote. There were twenty soloists in it and four different backdrops I made myself. My father built handmade table decorations. The program notes were printed on special paper that matched the cloth napkins, and the students all wore matching cowboy hats and bandanas. I thought out every detail in advance, from the tickets to the skirting on the risers. But I did every concert this way. When we were done, the audience often cried and gave us a standing ovation. Most of the time, when it ended, I would go home and slip into a dark room somewhere and fade away for a while.

During my second meeting with the counselor, she listened as I rambled on some more about my life growing up and my job. When I finished she said, "I'm thinking you're bipolar." I must've looked right through her because I clearly didn't know what bipolar meant and told her so. I said, "Well, I'm glad you know what's wrong, but I don't know what the hell bipolar means." She said I may have been more familiar with the term "manic depressive." She explained that I would crash after a concert because of manic cycling. She also said that would explain why I had difficulty creating some-times. It didn't explain the so-called "seizures," however. She told me there were a lot of different medications I could take to "even" me out so I wouldn't have so many ups and downs. She also explained that bipolar disorder has different levels, meaning it would worsen as I got older. It may also have explained why I never experi-enced depression as a child. She referred me to a psychi-atrist in Grand Rapids who would prescribe medication to treat my bipolar disorder. I set out to see her right away.

Multiple choice tests were never my thing. I would always read into them too much or forget which choice went with which bubble. I hate those things. So when I went to the psychiatrist, one can only guess what happened before I even met her: A one-thousand-question multiple-choice test arrived on my tabletop. I could feel a bullseye being placed on my chest. They put me in a room by myself and made me take that horrible test.

This test gave me more stress than any other I'd taken in my life. There were all kinds of double negatives to trick me and make sure I didn't lie. It would ask me the same thing in a different way to make sure I paid attention. I hated it. But I took it, fighting every urge to fall asleep instead. She didn't put a gold star on it or anything but I felt pretty good about it because it may have been the hardest test I ever took.

When I got into her office, she read over my enormous file and asked me just a few questions. She told me she felt I had bipolar disorder and wanted to start me on a medication called Zyprexa (olanzapine.) She also told me that Zyprexa would be the only medication I should need for bipolar and it would no longer be necessary to take Elavil. Like any other change in medication or a visitation with a new doctor, I soon touched base with my regular doctor to see how he felt about it. I wouldn't change anything without his approval. I wanted to make sure I could quit taking Elavil and begin the new medication. He agreed with her so I went off of the Elavil and began taking Zyprexa, watching my blood levels each week.

Back at work, I continued to produce the American Country Music Jamboree at the high school. I moved like I had a jet engine strapped to my back, teaching music and choreography, building sets, printing programs, deciding on the menu, painting, and yelling. When it came time for the show to happen, mania overtook me. The new medication seemed to work, though I would still cycle. Maybe not as often or as severe, but it would still happen. It happened on opening night in a big way.

It didn't happen much before, but during this particular show, I possessed quite a bit of irritability. At one point, some students who were supposed to be in the dining room were slacking off in another part of the building and I went off on them. I yelled at them, which I rarely did. I felt bad for it after I did it. In spite of my blow up, the revue came off without a hitch. I didn't crash afterwards, but I slowed down quite a bit. I didn't realize it at the time, but I still needed to get my life in order.

I felt pretty good at this point so I continued to work and plan for my next activity. Not long after the country revue, I went to see my counselor. She saw the show one night. I asked her what she thought because I knew she'd never seen one of our shows before. She loved it and praised the work I had done. I thanked her for the compliment. She said one person shouldn't be expected to do that much work. I said the students helped a lot, but I had difficulty completing it, since I arranged the music. She said she felt no one else could have done that. She said one person shouldn't expect that much from himself. I didn't know quite what she meant, but what she said next made sense.

"If you're going to continue to do this kind of work, you're going to have to learn to delegate. The reason you can do it now is because of your mania. You can't continue to count on that." Her statements seemed to be accurate. But as I was pretty stubborn, changing my work habits didn't come easy. I continued to work the same way and pushed myself harder when I needed to. The new medication worked quite well and I continued to prepare for the spring concert. I felt good. I didn't feel great, but I felt pretty good. I didn't give it a lot of thought then, but I don't know if I ever felt as though Zyprexa would be my final medication. I didn't realize that it can often take a long time to find the right medication to treat bipolar disorder. It sometimes takes more than one medication to manage a person's mood swings. But what did I know about it? I just figured they said you were bipolar, gave you a pill to take, and that would be the end of it. Now, I was learning about bipolar as I went, the hard way.

As the spring of 2002 breezed in, I still needed to do a lot of work. I took my show choir to my hometown every spring for an annual concert, the trip lasting an entire weekend. I needed to prepare for the Spring Choral Activities Concert which included the middle and high school choirs. I also needed to prepare the high school choir for their graduation song, and the middle school choir needed to prepare for eighth grade recognition. I had a lot on my plate, but I felt confident. I would just keep up an even pace and bring it all together. After all, I'd been teaching for more than fifteen years. I worked the same as I had every other year. I didn't worry about anything. What could go wrong?

All of my plans for spring fell into place just as they should. There were just a few weeks left in the school year. We just needed to prepare the concert choir and the middle school choir for the end of the year. I felt as though things were winding down fine. I hadn't forgotten anything. What could I forget? Perhaps what I'd forgotten about didn't pertain to work. Maybe I'd forgotten about those nasty old "seizures." Could they be coming back?

HELLO? ANYBODY HOME?

t sixteen years old I felt as though I knew everything. I felt I could do anything. I didn't need some adult telling me what to do. Just because they've lived a little longer and experienced more things doesn't make them an expert. I'd been driving almost a week so I could handle my father's car just fine.

It didn't matter that it didn't belong to me. I neglected to thank my father for turning over the car keys to me. He owed it to me. I deserved it because of the wonderful things I'd done for him growing up thus far. When he said "take it easy" it went in one ear and out the other, because with a week's driving experience, I knew what to do.

So off I went. I cruised nice and slow out of the driveway and down the road out of earshot. Then I kicked in the giant V8 and sucked down a little gasoline. I decided to clean out the fuel line a little. I'd been on these open roads all of my sixteen years and rolled over them having the time of my life. I picked up my friend Bill and let him in on the fun I'd stirred up.

Growing up in a very small town, most of my friends were lifelong. Bill fit that category. But I had a different relationship with him than my other friends. Time with Bill generally spelled trouble. I didn't always get caught when Bill and I were together, but it seems I often ended up in the possession of apples that weren't mine, or on the wrong end of a pumpkin smashing stick. Just the same, this seemed like a good day to see if he wanted to go for a ride.

We were in the car for about five minutes when things got interesting. The roads glazed up with newly fallen rain and someone else may have chosen to slow down. But I kept moving, rolling quickly over the pavement. We entered a curve and "the car" lost control, spun in circles a couple of times, and landed itself in the ditch. After what seemed like seconds, Bill's father came along, found us, and did me the favor of calling a tow truck. In a matter of minutes my little escapade became a town feature. I hoped all of the people there would keep this under their hats and that the kind man who loaned me the car, also known as "Dad," would never find out.

But coffee shops, gas stations, banks, and hardware stores are wonderful places to acquire information in a small town. Within twenty-four hours the news of my "outing" made a full circle and I suffered the inevitable consequences. My life spun out of control for the first time. But with a small price paid, I picked up the pieces and moved forward. As life went on, I would find things spinning out of control on occasion, but never to the point where I couldn't put the pieces back in order.

One mid-morning, I worked frantically to finish the year. It seemed like any other day at the middle school. Eighty kids were standing in front of me singing their hearts out preparing for yet another presentation when all of a sudden I got an old familiar taste in my mouth, metallic and strange. I'd tasted this before and I knew it would soon be followed by an intense head rush. I taught Erin, my daughter, in this class, and my wife, Debbie, taught in a nearby classroom. I told Erin to go get her mother to help me through the seizure. Soon the head rush came and after that I found myself at home asking unrelated questions. I became frustrated and went to see my doctor. He sent me in for blood work and found all my blood levels to be NORMAL! The Synthroid and Zyprexa levels were fine. Why the seizures? He didn't know, but he told me I could take some time off work if I wanted to. I wouldn't. No way in hell. I'd already taken off work in December and it almost drove me out of my mind. So I went back to work and finished out the week.

A few days later, during a normal weekend, things would change. Because Debbie and I were both teachers, we got invited to several graduation open houses in the spring. In our area, graduation parties are very popular and seeing as both Debbie and I taught so many kids, there were a bunch of them to go to. On this particular Sunday, we planned on going to several. We were just about to head out when I got the familiar taste in my mouth. This time, when I got the head rush I came out of it and started talking with a British accent. I don't recall any of it but my family remembered it well. I asked

Debbie, "What have you done with the children?" I spoke it in a wonderful British accent. Debbie described it as frightening. After a while, I stopped talking that way and became very confused, like the many times that had preceded this one. Debbie made the decision to go to an open house, but left me home with my oldest son. Though she was only gone for just a while, by the time she returned later that day, the event happened seven more times.

When Debbie described these "episodes" to me she said that during the one where I spoke with the British accent I looked right through her. This spooky episode frightened her. Our neighbor happened to be there when it took place and it scared the hell out of her as well. She and Debbie talked about it and the neighbor never told anyone. As a teacher, I felt a "mental illness" should be kept confidential. I lived in a small community where I taught more than a quarter of the students at the middle school and high school levels. With so many students and an opportunity for small town gossip, I thought it would be best to keep my health issues private. I was certain people would take a mental illness the wrong way and word would filter through the community. I was afraid I would be labeled as "crazy" even though I didn't feel that way.

During the course of the day, I continued having more of these episodes. Debbie kept close contact with my doctor and he planned to see me the next day to see if we could find some answers. For Debbie, the next day couldn't come soon enough. As the evening progressed, I calmed down enough to get some sleep, as did Debbie. But in the morning, the same thing started again. She couldn't handle me so she took me to the doctor's office as soon as she could. Up until that point, my doctor only heard of these "seizures" or "episodes." I described them to him many times. Now he would witness it.

But this day wasn't like the past. I grew tired of having so many of them and became angry. While in his office, I got the metallic taste in my mouth along with a head rush. Soon after that I punched the wall and yelled "This is bullshit!" I don't recall doing that but since my doctor, my counselor, Debbie, and several wide-eyed office assistants were there to witness it, I guess I have to agree with them. My doctor turned to Debbie and said, "Is this what happens every time?" And she said, "No! He's never done that before!" I generally didn't have a violent bone in my body. But for the remainder of the day, I showed a lot of aggression.

As a young man I wasn't considered a very big guy. As I've gotten older, I've picked up some weight, a little height, and my shoulders have broadened. I'm now six-foot-two and weigh about 225 pounds. When someone of my size isn't thinking straight and becomes agitated, it's best to get them under control. My doctor gave me a shot to calm me down and put me in his office to rest. But I wasn't calm. I was up and down and remained irritated the whole time. Debbie stayed with me to try and keep me calm, with little success.

Before the day ended, I went to the hospital for observation. While there, I behaved like an ass. I yelled and swore and pleaded with Debbie to "get me the fuck out of here!" The doctor gave me enough tranquilizers to calm a horse, but they didn't work for me. I became very manic and nothing seemed to get me under control. After what felt like forever, I calmed down and the seizures stopped. The doctor decided to let me go home the next day. He also decided to put me back on Elavil. I'd never had seizures or episodes while taking Elavil, so he prescribed it as sort of a safety net. My doctor explained that while he agreed to let me go home, I needed to take two weeks off of work to rest. I wasn't happy about it because there were so many things to do before the end of the year. But the more I argued, the more I realized I didn't have a choice. Later in the day we got a call from my sister-in-law saying she and her husband were flying in to visit for a few days. They were coming in to keep an eye on me and keep me out of trouble, but I welcomed them anyway.

When they arrived, they found me in the garage building a new post for the mailboxes at the end of the driveway. I was supposed to be resting and when they asked me about it, I said I *was* resting, but I needed to get this done. My brother-in-law shook his head and walked into the house. I had an old car that I tinkered with in my spare time and since I couldn't drive for two weeks, any time I wanted to go somewhere, my brother-in-law would put the top down and take me for a ride. It worked out well because he got to drive a pretty cool car and I got out of the house. My sister-in-law kept busy in the house by making sure I didn't reorganize the spice rack or build new silverware inserts for the drawers. She also got me to all of my blood draws and doctor's appointments, because there were quite a few and I had trouble keeping them straight.

Debbie worked during the day and needed them there to look after me. One day I couldn't stand being cooped up anymore, so I asked my brother-in-law to drive me to the high school to visit my students. In the back of my mind, I knew Debbie would give me hell for it but I couldn't stand being gone so long at the end of the year and did it anyway. When I got there, I found them working hard and the substitute doing a great job. They were all glad to see me. I enjoyed seeing them, but I didn't stay long. I pretended to need something out of my desk. It set my mind at ease to see them doing so well and I rested better at home after going. But I still needed answers. Why was my health and my life such a mess? Why did the seizures come back and what were they anyway? Maybe the doctor would have some answers.

A state of confusion came over my doctor. He knew that if the seizures came back once, they could come back again. He'd never seen anything like them before. After he witnessed them, he told us that they were out of his league. I respected my doctor's willingness to refer me to someone else when he didn't know how to treat me. This time he decided to go straight to the top. When the school year came to an end, he sent me to the Mayo Clinic for a psychiatric evaluation and a wealth of other tests. I looked forward to hearing from the Mayo Clinic.

Nobody hopes they can go to the Mayo Clinic someday. It's not on anyone's bucket list. When one gets referred to the Mayo Clinic, it means no one else can figure out what's wrong. But for me, going to the Mayo Clinic was kind of cool. First of all, my parents took care of our kids, so Debbie and I got to go away together for a few days, which didn't often happen. They also let us use their brand-new car so we didn't have to drive our gas guzzling conversion van all the way out there.

When we arrived, we found an unbelievable facility and I knew I would be in good hands. Right away, I gave blood samples. I give blood samples all the time and I hate it because my veins tend to roll. The nurse misses them and they end up poking me about five times before they hit a vein. I often come out of there covered in tape. This time was different. The nurse just grabbed my arm, wiped it down, and stuck the needle in. She got it on the first try, no problem. She proceeded to fill all the vials, then said, "Have a nice day!" I told her it often takes five or six times before they can hit my veins. She said "I've seen two-hundred patients already, and it's only 8:00." I guess if you do something often enough, you're bound to get good at it.

They scheduled an electroencephalogram. I always just say EEG because it's too hard to say Electroencephalogram. It's used to measure electrical activity in your brain. Little suction cups are attached to your scalp and connected to a computer. The computer measures the electrical activity and records it with wavy lines on paper. Health professionals can then measure seizure activity. It's best to go in tired because they prefer that the patient sleep during the test. Luckily, I could sleep for a little while. The test showed no evidence of seizure activity. That came as good news, but confusing, knowing my treatment history.

Later in my visit to the Mayo Clinic, I saw a neurologist. I waited for a while to see him. When he came in he looked like Frank Zappa's brother. He didn't look like any other neurologist I'd ever seen. He asked me a lot of questions, went through my very thick file and examined me physically. He tested my reflexes, looked in my eyes with a light, and made me sniff some wintergreen. He didn't give me a diagnosis of any kind at the time. His notes would be sent to my doctor at a later date. He did mention that Zyprexa might not be the best medication for bipolar disorder, however. I began to understand why the "seizures" occurred. I started to feel as though whatever they were, happened because of the wrong medication.

When we left his office, we walked to the subway en route to see a psychiatrist. But, before I saw the psychiatrist, I would have to take some tests. Multiple-choice tests. This time I took TWO! One contained a thousand questions and the other, five hundred. I tried to stay awake as I took the tests. I also took a math test, which I failed, and several others. There were blocks of different shapes and I tried to put them together the way I thought they fit best. I felt comfortable with it, but it took me a long time. With so many ideas scurrying around in my head, I found it difficult to come up with the best choice. No answer I gave could be right or wrong. The test administrator told me to "just make the most logical choice." I saw so many different shapes and designs in those damned blocks. If it weren't for the time limit, I'd still be sitting there. But over time, I made choices and came up with designs that were creative and pleasing to the eye.

Debbie went with me when I saw the psychiatrist because she could help me explain the "seizures" a little better. Plus, I needed her to help me remember everything he said. I started at the beginning of my journey and told him pretty much everything. I told him about my childhood and my job. I told him of the cycling, mania, depression, and "seizures." The whole time I spoke he sat in his chair with his elbows on his desk and his hands under his chin. He listened to us and said "Mm-hm, Mm-hm" as I thought he might.

When I describe my experiences, I sometimes sugar-coat things a little, so Debbie quickly chimed in and made sure things didn't sound better than they were. She made sure he understood the severity of every symptom, but still let me tell my own story. When I described myself, he said, "You seem to be correctly diagnosed with bipolar disorder." When I spoke in detail about the seizures and told him about the metallic taste and the head rush, followed by confusion, he looked at me without batting an eye and said, "That's a type of manic episode. It's not uncommon." Debbie and I were flabbergasted! All this time I'd been treated for seizures and in a matter of minutes this man told me about a different form of manic episode! Most people get excited or perhaps go off on a rampage. Sometimes they spend money they don't have or do things they later regret. I get a bad taste in my mouth, have a head rush and forget things. I'd never done anything like anyone else before in my life. Why should I have manic episodes the same as everyone else?

No doctor in my area ever heard of this type of manic episode before, but this particular doctor treated many cases like mine. He suggested a different medication than Zyprexa. He spoke of Depakote (divalproex sodium) and told me he didn't think it would be necessary to take Elavil with Depakote. Depakote, he told me, would control the manic episodes fine by itself.

We stayed in a hotel while we were at the Mayo Clinic. After my visit to the psychiatrist, I went back to my room and found the light blinking on the phone. I found a message on it from my doctor at home. He wanted me to call and tell him what the psychiatrist said. He didn't want to wait a few days for the report so I called and filled him in. When I spoke with him, I heard relief in his voice when he found out the cause of my seizure problem.

Now I would start a new chapter of my life. I suffered from manic episodes that were so severe I would need medication to control them. My moods were cycling so often that I needed to control those as well. A stroke history left scar tissue on my brain, but so far, the scars had no other effect on me. Medication helped my non-functioning thyroid gland. I also took medication for a hiatal hernia and suffered from intense heartburn. But other than that, things were good. I would start this new medication and go on with my life. I felt lucky that the medication change would take place during the summer when I wasn't working so I could go on and off the drugs gradually until the levels were right. Bring on the Depakote!

LEARN TO LIVE WITH IT

*A*fter a mind boggling trip to the Mayo Clinic, I would put all of my new knowledge to work. The "seizures" I'd been having were really manic episodes. With the right medication, they should be easy to treat. The doctors at the Mayo Clinic made me feel kind of "normal" when they noted that I was one of millions of people living with bipolar. What a great feeling! Driving home from Minnesota to Michigan with Debbie, I looked forward to a new start. I felt good about using the next few weeks to try a new medication and looked forward to going back to work in the fall as a revitalized teacher with fresh ideas. I started implementing the new plan.

Changing medication is a bitch. This change would be no exception. I drained all of the Zyprexa out of my system and began adding the Depakote. It took a few weeks to get the dosage right and I'm pretty sure that during that time everyone saw me as a pain in the ass.

My cycles were numerous, random, and drastic. I started a lot of projects and left a lot of things unfinished. I talked all the time and ran out of ideas before I finished my sentences. But soon, we found the right balance and I evened out. I concentrated and functioned quite well. I spent the summer getting used to the "new me" and looked for enough of the "old me" in there for people to recognize. I also needed enough of my creative side to do my job. I hoped Depakote wouldn't keep me from thinking creatively.

Riding beats walking. It beats walking so much that I found myself desperate for an automobile. My cousin blazed up the driveway in one of Chevrolet's worst mistakes: a 1976 Chevrolet Vega GT. But this time a "For Sale" sign covered the window. What a lucky day! At nineteen years old, I didn't know about the reputation of the Vega GT. I only saw a sleek little car with bright orange paint, custom wheels, and a for sale sign!

I soon possessed a bright orange Vega GT that needed paint, a tune-up, new brakes, and much more. Mostly interested in the paint job, I decided '73 Corvette Yellow would be the shade to cover the car. Bright orange and red stripes over the trunk and down the sides dressed it up nice. Everywhere I went people looked at the brightest, most colorful car in the county.

Despite the new paint job, I found it still didn't run right. It needed a tune-up. The brakes still made noise when I pushed on the pedal and the "Check Engine" light shined proudly from the instrument panel. The fact is, beneath that bright new paint job, the Vega was still just a Vega.

Several side effects went along with Depakote that I didn't like. I suffered from slight confusion and couldn't concentrate. I would have a little trouble stringing words together and finishing sentences, but I wasn't bothered by it much because I'd dealt with rapid thought for so long this wasn't a big issue. I also gained weight quickly. I spent my first thirty years thin as a rail. I would hear the joke, "If you stood sideways and stuck out your tongue, you'd look like a zipper!" From age thirty to forty I sported an average weight. When I went on Depakote, I went from 200 pounds to 250 instantly. Thank you, Depakote.

But in spite of the challenges, as the summer of 2002 progressed I became more and more comfortable with Depakote. I played in a rock band for several years and had an upcoming gig. This would be a good opportunity for me to pilot the new drug. I would play a four-hour show with nonstop music. Since we were a small local group, we set up, played music, and tore down. It would be a chance for me to test my memory and stamina. As the night progressed, I got a few stares from the other guys in the band because I often made mistakes and forgot lyrics, even though they were right in front of me. I made mistakes on "Proud Mary" and other songs. "Proud Mary?" I'd played that song so many times I should've been able to play it in my sleep.

I needed time to adjust to the Depakote. I needed to practice my music or mellow out, or something. When I spoke to my doctor about it, he said Depakote would have side effects and I should tolerate them. "*Tolerate* them?" I said. "I can *tolerate* jock itch!" He just laughed and told me that if the medication helped bipolar and stopped the manic episodes, then I should try it for a while. So I did.

I used Depakote for about three years. During that time, the manic episodes seemed to be under control. However, after about a month of taking the drug, I noticed slight tremors. If I held a coffee cup, it would shake in my hand. I tried holding my hand out in front of me and noticed it trembling in the air. As a conductor, this presented a problem. When I held my baton out in front of me it started to shake. School would start up again in less than a month and my baton shook when I held it in front of me. I needed to put a stop to this unwanted side effect.

I did everything I could to stop the tremors. I went to the doctor and he said that he couldn't do anything about it. I practiced like crazy trying to even out my conducting. But nothing worked. So I started the school year with a shaky baton. I compensated for it by holding the students at attention for shorter amounts of time. At the end of songs I'd cut them off sooner and get the baton down faster. I even stopped using the baton a lot, conducting with just my hands, but I still noticed the trembling. I know the students noticed it too, but I don't recall any of them ever saying anything.

One day while working with the concert choir at the high school, the principal came into my classroom. She said she needed to see me right then. Someone came in to watch my class for a minute and she took me out in the parking lot. At the high school, the drug dogs would make random visits. On this particular day they sniffed out my car. They needed me to open it so they could search it. I knew I didn't have any medication in my car and felt embarrassed. After the search, they found a small bottle with a few Ibuprofen tablets in the glove box. I got hauled out of class and embarrassed in front of the whole school because of a few Ibuprofen? It didn't make sense.

Later, the principal talked to me about it in her office and she said she wasn't worried. She knew me long enough and well enough to know that I wouldn't have drugs or alcohol in my car. She talked to the K-9 officer about it and she said that if a person takes a lot of prescription medication it can seep out of their pores into the seat cushions. That, compounded with the few Ibuprofen, seemed to be enough to alert the dog. I'd never heard of this before but I never carried Ibuprofen or any other medication in my car again.

This made me realize that I needed to be discreet about my illness and my medications. I lived and worked in a small town where people talked. If they found out, people might blow my "mental illness" out of proportion, an ongoing fear I had. Since the mini-stroke in 1998, I often said I suffered from complications of that. It kept people happy and I didn't have to go into any detail. I continued to work and tried hard to produce excellence with the choral program. I began to slow down at this point, but said very little about it and continued my usual routine.

I never got much sleep. I created my best while

everyone else slept. Depakote didn't change that one bit. I'd go to bed at eleven o'clock like everyone else and be wide awake in a couple of hours finding things to do. If I got five hours of sleep in a night I celebrated. I often told myself I could always make up for it the next night, but I knew in the back of my mind I wouldn't catch up. When I was manic all the time it didn't matter, but now that the mood swings were under control, lack of sleep started to burn me out. The days were long and I couldn't get kick-started in the morning. Because I didn't sleep most of the night, I would often crash about the time I needed to start my day.

I taught two middle school choirs first thing in the morning. Who needed my attention more than a class of 80 seventh- and eighth-graders? I did everything I could to be on my game for them. I picked out exciting music. I taught choreography. I pushed myself as hard as I could to keep things engaging. I taught the high school choir at 10:30 in the morning and found it to be my perfect time of day. I worked very well at this time and so did the students.

We accomplished a lot and the program became very well known in the community. By the afternoon, however, I started to slow down. I taught a guitar class that was decidedly laid-back compared to the high intensity of the school choir, and did planning at the end of the day. I often found myself counting the minutes until that plan period, not because I didn't like my job, but because of lack of sleep.

I talked to my doctor about the possibility of medication to help me sleep and we decided that with all of the other medications in place, that it wouldn't be a good idea. So I worked my butt off and slept when I could. I gained weight from the Depakote but it evened out my mood swings and helped me do my job. I didn't like the way the Depakote made me feel, though. I felt slow, clod-dish, and controlled. Creativity didn't come as easily as before. I'd heard a lot about how many people with bipolar disorder didn't take their medication regularly, didn't take it properly, or would quit taking it at all, after a while. This didn't surprise me because medication often makes one feel different. Some people don't feel like they're the same person. For me, I didn't have as much energy and couldn't create easily. At one time, I could write songs in my sleep and create things by the hour. Now, ideas came slowly. I didn't always like how I felt. I knew, however, that if I didn't take my medication, I'd have manic episodes that were unlike most people with bipolar disorder, and my family and I wouldn't be able to cope with them. I also knew that bipolar disorder worsens with age. I figured if I didn't take my medication the right way, I would be very hard to deal with later in life.

So I took Depakote and remained easy to get along with. At least I felt easy to get along with. I still didn't get much sleep. My moods still cycled, although they weren't as severe as they'd once been. I continued to work. I produced shows, traveled with my groups, and strived to be a good father and husband. I remained concerned about weight gain and cholesterol, but all of the dieting in the world didn't seem to fight the wrath of Depakote. I felt sluggish from the drug and pretty fat. I felt as though a medication change would help me. I waited, though. My doctor thought that changing medications would be a big undertaking and we should wait until summer when I didn't teach. He also wanted to do some research to find the right drug or combination of drugs. I continued to take Depakote. Although there were health concerns, my support group helped me through this difficult time in my life.

IT TAKES AN ARMY

We loved being around the people who knew us the best and enjoyed us the most. Being with family was the perfect pastime. We went to see Debbie's aunt and uncle and they decided to go to a community building on this lazy Sunday so the kids could play for a while.

We arrived at the building and soon the kids were at play, laughing, running, and jumping around happily. Some were playing basketball, some were playing dodgeball, some were skipping rope, and some were just playing. My kids were quite little at the time and needed a lot of "guidance" because they were so young, but also because sports wasn't our area of expertise and they didn't have much experience. That's where Gary stepped in.

Uncle Gary decided that my two oldest children, Michael and Erin, should line up at one end of the gym and race to the other end. They were both excited about the idea and stood on the line as he instructed them to. He went through all of the antics that a *good coach would. He set his stopwatch, put his hand in the air, and prepared to shout out "ON YOUR MARK!" But when he looked down at the two young children, they were standing on the line grinning at each other, holding hands. He laughed out loud at the two competitors when he realized neither of them were in a race before and the brother and sister were such good friends that beating one another hadn't crossed their minds.*

Uncle Gary did what any good coach would do. He explained the idea behind a race to them and told them how to prepare for it. He even showed them the finish line and short-ened the distance a little. There were no losers in that race. When you have as tight a family bond as we did, everyone comes up winning.

When my kids were little they would come to me with a broken toy and say "Daddy fix?" They'd look up at me with their big brown or hazel eyes and I would just melt. Then I'd look down at the mangled piece of plastic in their hands and my wheels began to turn. My kids didn't often break toys. They tended to take good care of everything. I felt a strong responsibility to try as hard as I could to reassemble a toy that should have been thrown in the trash. I would use a solder gun to heat and repair cracks in plastic. I would make wheels and spare parts out of wood or rubber or whatever I could to repair the broken toy, as well as repaint and replace parts. Soon I would give it back and say, "There you go, as good as new." A smile and a hug was the only repayment I ever got and the only one I ever needed.

As time went by, things would continue to break. Toys, computers, guitars, cars, and even an occasional heart. They still came to me for help. "Dad, can you fix this?" Later in life, the wheels didn't turn as fast, but the task would still get done. This was my place. It still is, and I hope it always will be. But I also needed repairs from time to time. Not just from my doctor, but from a loving family. I *always* got it. It may have been something small, like my son coming to me and saying, "How are you doing today, Dad?" Now how did a fifteen-year-old kid know when a man struggled, coming to him in the middle of the day just to give him an extra nudge to help him along? He saw my emotional battles more than the younger kids and just seemed to know. Being a soft-hearted soul, he was very intuitive.

When I struggled to get out of bed in the morning, my daughter would sometimes come into my room and say, "It's time to get up now, Dad." A few minutes later, she'd repeat the process until I got to my feet and moved about my day. Why did a fourteen-year-old know what to do without being told? At times, I would struggle to get projects done at work, particularly involving building or being creative. What made a kid show up at the school and just take a hammer in hand and help at a time when I needed it most? Somehow they all knew.

When you're a kid, you're a kid. That's all there is to it. I said that before, but this time the context is different. This time I'm talking about three kids who grew up with a bipolar parent. They supported me and followed me on my journey because they saw me this way all of their lives. They watched me transform from a full blown "busy kid" to someone with deep depression, anger, and cycles of highs and lows, to someone with some pretty heavy manic episodes. But through it all, they were always loved, and they knew it. They loved me back, and I knew it.

I think honesty became the key to our success. Debbie and I decided that we would tell them everything we knew about my illness as it progressed and fill them in whenever we learned something new or if something changed. We also told them why I never discussed my illness with anyone. We told them they could each choose a close friend to talk about it with if they wanted. We didn't do that until they were a little older and I believe they all shared it with a friend. Since they've all become young adults, they've opened up about it a little more, but when they were young they respected my privacy.

My oldest son Michael has been an artist all of his life. From a very young age we watched him take a pencil into his hand and create things that we couldn't under-stand until he finished. We've watched him paint, build and do digital artwork that we marveled at. At the age of eight or nine he used a drawing program on the computer to create different shapes and colors. He drew a few shapes and soon they would disappear. Then he would draw a few more and they too would disappear. This went on for a little while when he turned to me and said, "Watch this!" He gave one click of the mouse and all of the shapes he'd been working on joined together to form one beautiful picture. We were amazed that he knew how to do that. An eight-year-old did things with that program that most adults never knew were possible. Through the years, we've listened to him try to explain things to us, struggling to find the words, but when he showed us his completed project, it all made perfect sense. He told me he sleeps very little and creates deep into the night. Like me, he has periods of time when he can't create, but when his creative juices are flowing they seem to overflow. As he has grown older, he's struggled somewhat with anxiety and depression, but has been able to keep it under control without medication thus far.

My middle child is my daughter, Erin. At the age of two, we took her to the beach one blustery afternoon. My father happened to be there to capture her on film. She sang the entire Brahms Lullaby from memory on the beach that day. Even at the young age of two, she made music. When she reached middle school, there would be a thump when she entered the house and her backpack hit the floor. We could hear footsteps as she ran through the house. When she reached the piano, the music would start. It would continue until bedtime every night throughout her middle and high school years. As she got older, she earned countless solos and parts in plays and became a skilled musician. As time went by, she earned her bachelor's degree in vocal performance. Erin's creativity runs a different course, but her ability to handle a full schedule and juggle multiple activities is amazing. Sometimes, though, she will drift away and slow down for a while. She often goes through periods of extreme sadness, having trouble fighting off the tears. After a little rejuvenation, she'll return, ready to take on the world again. She married a man with three children who live with them and now has a child of her own. Finding ways to manage a large family so suddenly has been a challenge for her. She does whatever she can to keep it all together.

When my youngest child, David, was quite small, he needed to do a science project. All science projects required a solution to a problem. We visited the drive-through window of the bank many times, watching the money carriers traveling from the car to the bank and back through transparent tubes. David wondered whether the machine sucked the tube to the bank or blew it to the bank. So, he built a miniature bank with plastic tubes and miniature money carriers. With my help, he used an air compressor to blow the carrier through the tube and a vacuum to suck it through. I don't remember what he decided the results were, but I learned that David wasn't the type of kid to soak pennies in four different brands of ketchup to see which one made them cleaner. His ideas, even at a young age, were much deeper. Sometimes he gets a lot of ideas in his head at once and it's difficult to keep them straight, but he works hard to organize his thoughts and seems to function quite well. He now has his bachelor's degree in film and has been working diligently to keep his ideas and creativity in order. He is an independent film editor and works around the clock, just like his father. I worry that mania will catch up to him and depression may overcome him, but he's been able to manage it thus far.

All three of our children have become very creative young adults and have grown to be quite skilled at what they do. We're proud of their accomplishments. Because of my medical history, all three of them need to watch for symptoms of bipolar disorder and other mental illnesses. Because bipolar is hereditary, Debbie and I have made sure that they are aware of it and watch for any signs that they may need to seek medical attention. Because people with mental illnesses often don't want to accept it or deal with it, we continue to monitor them and remind them of my struggles with bipolar. We feel that if they develop a mental illness of any kind, or have one currently, it's best to have it diagnosed and treated as soon as possible. It's probable that if they begin treatment earlier, their symptoms might not be as severe.

There's one person who's been through more hell than anyone through all of this, and that's Debbie. At twenty-one years old, she saw me as a kind and caring man with a new career at his feet and a TON of energy. I worked hard, played hard, and made life romantic and fun. I kept things interesting and lighthearted. I proposed right away so I could be with her forever.

She accepted my proposal and when I gave her an engagement ring, she tackled me. I stumbled over a bed frame and tore open my toe. It bled a river and neither of us cared. We just laughed, cried and began our journey together. But we didn't realize that through sickness and in health, richer or poorer, until death do us part, I would become a different man than the one she married. But she stayed. Through all of it, she stayed and supported me. She helped me through countless medication changes and mood swings. When the person one loves slips into a deep depression and nothing that is said or done can bring them out of it, how easy would it be to walk away? But Debbie didn't. When the manic episodes happened and I looked right through her, screaming obscenities at her in the hospital, she stayed. She stayed, supported me, and loved me unconditionally.

When I became obsessed with my job and worked all of the time, I could always count on her to be there. She came to my shows and videotaped them. She sewed costumes and did the girls' hair. She even did a guy's hair once. It was greasy and gross, but she did it. During our annual dinner show, she came and organized the dining room and taught the kids how to wait tables. She helped design sets and decorate for concerts no matter how I behaved, and it wasn't always pretty. It never caused us to lose our relationship but we came close on a few occasions. I nearly lost her a few times because of my careless and almost irate behavior. I think that in her heart, she knew that I couldn't do it alone, and I couldn't. I needed her support so much that I'm sure I wouldn't have made it to where I am without her. I couldn't have worked and changed medications without her help. I couldn't have gotten out of bed and gotten to work on time each day without her encouragement. I might not have made the most logical choices without her guidance. Unconditional love is the hardest kind to find. I feel like the luckiest man alive because I've had Debbie loving me unconditionally for more than thirty-six years. I believe every person struggling with bipolar disorder needs a strong support group. Fortunately, I had one in place from the beginning.

I never felt as though my parents and siblings were as understanding as my wife and children. They weren't unsupportive, they just didn't understand bipolar disorder and weren't around me enough to notice the problems as they occurred. Bipolar disorder is very difficult to diagnose and I believe it's at least as difficult to explain. When I learned of bipolar disorder in 2001 I said, "What the hell is that?" I wasn't alone in my unawareness of the illness. When diagnosed with bipolar disorder, I had a long "seizure" history, along with a ministroke that I'd been hospitalized for, in addition to a hiatal hernia and hypothyroidism. So when I told my family I'd been diagnosed with bipolar disorder I think their internal response may have been, "Oh, God, what the hell has he come down with now?"

In a way, I can't blame them. But my parents showed their support in other ways. My parents were the Shelby Choral Department's biggest fans. My dad helped me build sets and built handmade table decorations for the dinner revue that were beautiful. He made twenty a year for around sixteen years. When the choir came to their town on tour, my mother made food for all of them. She promoted concerts in her hometown more than anyone could be expected to. Both of them came early to concerts, stayed late, and the props that my father built were stunning. It helped take some of the stress out of my very busy schedule.

My Dad was born on a farm in Onekama, Michigan, and lived there almost all of his life. When he got married, he bought some land from my grandfather and built a house next door. I looked up to my father because I didn't know many people with more talent. He didn't possess musical ability, but when it came to getting something done, almost anything, he could figure it out. He could draw, paint, build, create, and think better than most anyone I knew. He liked to work on cars, which I loved. He never seemed too tired to do a project when he got home from a hard day at work. I loved helping him with his projects. He was a good, hard-working man with a lot of ideas. I think that some of my creative genes came from him. We spent a lot of time working side by side on projects through the years, and I believe that some of my life decisions were difficult for him to process. As time went by, he grew more and more accepting of them and became one of my strongest supporters.

I've never known a time when my Mom wasn't working. She worked at a hotel when we were young and at the school as an assistant after that. When I got a little older, she worked in the office the county road commission. But that's not the kind of work I'm referring to. Ever since I can remember, and to this day, I can't think of a time when she wasn't picking something up, brushing something off, washing something, cooking something, or putting something away. She made a huge list of people that she sent birthday cards and other holiday cards to each month and seldom missed an event. At ninety-one years young, she still sends cards to a long list of people. If she came over to visit, she always brought a treat for everyone there. Sometimes I think that my bursts of energy may have come from her. She never seemed to tire of doing good things for others and I'm glad to have her support and kindness.

I believe that people with bipolar disorder deserve a good support system, but what I've come to learn is that it shouldn't stop there. I think the families of people with bipolar disorder need help, understanding, and support as well. They're often affected by the disorder just as much as the person who has it. That is one of the reasons we were so open with our children when they were growing up. It's also why we let them open up to a friend about it. Debbie confided in a few friends along the way, as well, and so did I. Any time I opened up with a friend about it, I told them I didn't talk to people about it much because of my teaching profession and that I'd rather they not say anything. Debbie did the same thing. I don't know if anyone ever broke that confidence, but we lived in a small town and it never got back to us.

Debbie also read a lot about bipolar disorder and acquired a lot of information that way. I waited for her to read a book and then she would tell me everything she read. That system worked quite well...for me. We got a lot of good information from books. Some came from research and some came from testimony. We found usefulness in all of it, but mainly we learned to keep the whole family informed.

We were certain, based on what we'd learned from doctors, counselors, the internet, and books that bipolar disorder would not go away. We also knew that any medications that I would take for bipolar disorder might keep it under control, but they wouldn't cure it. There *is* no "cure" for bipolar disorder. There are ways to control it with medication, but no way to stop it. I found that even when taking medications to control bipolar, symptoms still happened. They weren't as severe but they were still there. That's why I needed a strong support system in place. I needed loving people in my life. They needed to be people who would understand me and believe in me no matter what. With the help of Debbie and the kids, I could continue down a path that would make me feel useful and successful, which wasn't always easy. The path would have to change, but my family would help me identify and deal with change when it happened. That's all I ever needed. I called them my Army. They were behind me, helping me fight a constant battle to stay well. My Army was small, but they were powerful and they were always at my side.

13

LIFE IS A THEATRE PRODUCTION

*I*n 2005, I started slowing down and felt that Depakote wasn't working for me as well as it had been. I talked to my doctor about it and he told me about a newer medication with the pleasing side effect of weight loss. Topamax (topiramate) seemed like a wonder drug. I said "Sign me up!" I couldn't wait to try a new medication and after a little research, Topamax sounded like the right alternative. I found out that I could lose around fifty pounds. Plus, I might have more energy than I did on Depakote and the tremors would go away. Bring it on!

I've said it before, but changing medication is a bitch! I dialed back the Depakote slowly and began taking Topamax. I needed to have my blood levels checked each week to determine the right medication level in my system. It took about a month until everything evened out. By the end of the summer, I felt great. I dropped fifty pounds right away. The tremors went away and my energy increased. I could hold my baton steady and conduct smoothly and freely. Looking forward to the new school year, I felt I'd found a new me! I bought new clothes to start the school year because my old clothes didn't fit. I rearranged my classrooms so the students could have a new start, just like me. I redesigned my office to make it more efficient. I felt just a *little* manic and that seemed like a good thing.

Just like every other medication, there were side effects. Sometimes when we would walk together, Debbie pointed out that I often curled my hands in. I would tuck my thumbs in and make a loose fist. It wasn't a big deal but I'd never done it before. She also noticed that I would sometimes grind my teeth. Again, not a big deal, but something new. I talked to my doctor about it and he reduced my Topamax level just a little and those effects went away. The school year started, which meant I would get to take Topamax for a real test drive. I started teaching and everything went fine. At first.

I started working like a fool again, rehearsing as hard as ever. Being quite the storyteller, I could make a story from almost anything and somehow weave it into my lesson. In roughly mid-September, I set out to do just that. All eighty-five concert choir students were focused on me as I told one of my many stories. I got somewhere in the middle of it when my thoughts jumbled up. It became hard to complete sentences and stay focused. I got overly emotional about the topic, couldn't keep my thoughts straight, and began to tear up. It didn't go well at all. I was completely pissed off. I spoke to my doctor and he said he believed it to be the medication but didn't know quite what to do. Why couldn't I find a damned medication that worked?

A new psychologist had recently come to the building and I went to see him. I met with him and immediately found him likable. He played the guitar and liked Hendrix, Eric Clapton and many others. He kept a calm and cool disposition. I found him easy to talk to. He liked old cars and loved my Mustang. In addition, he was a hell of a doctor and did a lot of tests on me that I'd never done. I retook the thousand-question multiple choice test, but this time he showed me how he graded it.

He showed me why there were so many double negatives and why they were useful. He told me that the Topamax would do a good job, but that I would need another medication to act as a mood stabilizer to keep my thoughts together and to keep me from being overly emotional. He prescribed a light dosage of Abilify (aripiprizole). I felt comfortable with his choice and believed that Abilify would be the answer to my problems. So I took it.

Soon after taking Abilify I got a very dry mouth. It became so dry that I couldn't swallow. I talked to my doctor and he cut my dosage down. Right away the problem disappeared and I could concentrate again. I've heard many people refer to Topamax as "Stupimax" and I understand that many people who have taken it have had trouble concentrating. I believe taking Abilify in combination with Topamax helped me avoid that undesirable side effect. Another side effect of Topamax is that it makes soda pop taste awful. Any carbonated beverage tasted terrible for me while taking Topamax, so if one is a hardcore soda drinker, they may want to consider another medication.

I started taking the combination of Topamax and Abilify in 2005. It continued to work for many years. Not all combinations of medications are right for everyone because not all people who suffer from bipolar disorder have the same symptoms. But this particular combination of medications helped me to function for quite some time.

I now took Elavil, Topamax, and Abilify to control my bipolar disorder. I had a strong choral group at the high school and I worked as hard as I could to keep the choirs on top. In 2006 the show choir won a thirty-school talent competition. Meanwhile, the concert choir performed a Beatles Revue that impressed our local audiences. In the morning, before I went to work, I would often get ready and then fall asleep in a chair until Debbie told me to get up and go. When I got home at the end of the day (or night, when I worked extra long hours) I would crash in a chair for a while to regain enough energy to function. But every day I got up and kept moving. Some days, when I would cycle into mania, I could get by on little or no sleep. Other days I wasn't so lucky.

Even with medication I would still cycle. Debbie could always recognize the mania because I would wiggle my feet. They wouldn't wiggle just a little. My feet would almost shake the whole room as I sat in my chair wiggling them. When I was manic, I couldn't sit still. I would often find something to do with all of the extra energy. Trying to be still didn't work at all. I tried to find something useful to do because if I became manic, that meant I would crash soon. Debbie always watched over me when I became manic (and she still does) because she knew that depression would follow.

I should've known it too, but recognizing mania hasn't always been my strong suit. Part of the reason for this may be that I happen to *like* mania. I like feeling I can accomplish anything or feeling like I'm *really* happy and excited. I like running around the house with a thousand ideas in my head. The problem was, and still is, that I seldom completed many of the tasks I started while manic. I'm not sure if students could tell that my moods changed frequently or not. I became very good at disguising the mood swings. For me, being bipolar meant being a good actor. I'd been a performer all of my life, so acting "up" when I needed to was easy.

That ability is not always a good thing, though. It would often irritate Debbie because I would dread going out to an event. I didn't want to go at all. Not being a drinker meant that I would be hanging out with a bunch of drinkers at a party who were laughing at things that I didn't think were as funny as they did. I complained a lot about going. But after being dragged there, I laughed, told jokes, and pretended to have a good time. It would drive her crazy. She would listen to me whine about going somewhere for hours, including on the ride there. Then when we arrived I would turn on the "party animal." I figured as long as I had to go, I might as well have a good time. Also, once you turn on the performer it's a little hard to turn him off.

———

I could feel the heat coming from the lights as I sat in darkness backstage. In full makeup, I waited to make my entrance. It was opening night and soon the audience would see "The Lion" for the first time. I may have been more excited to play this part than any other. "The Lion" in The Wizard of Oz *was one of my favorite characters of all time and I felt lucky to land the part in the beautiful one-hundred-year-old Ramsdell Theatre in Manistee, Michigan. To make things even more exciting, the famous James Earl Jones came to opening night!*

The time came for me to jump out on the stage! When I did, I could hear the audience gasp and then laugh as I went through all of the antics I prepared for "The Lion" to perform. I enjoyed becoming someone else and having all of those eyes watch me as they enjoyed the performance. At the end of the play, I remained excited because I would get to perform it five more times. It meant wearing the hottest costume I'd ever put on, sticking a prosthetic nose on my face, and wearing uncomfortable makeup. But it also gave me the opportunity to become someone I wasn't for a little while. During that time I could dance, sing, laugh, perform, and make people happy.

On a beautiful Sunday afternoon we performed our matinee, which would be our final performance. Afterwards, the cast went out in the audience and found many of them to be children. A lot of those children came dressed as characters from The Wizard of Oz. *We took dozens of pictures and signed nearly as many autographs. Then "The Lion" went backstage and transformed back into Dana.*

After a lot of scrubbing and shampooing, I returned to my normal self and went with my family to get ice cream at a little shop along the river in beautiful downtown Manistee. As we sat at a picnic table enjoying our well earned treat, I looked over at the next table and noticed a little girl whom I'd just taken a picture with at the theatre. I approached her and said, "Do I look familiar to you?" and she shook her head as if to say "No." Without my makeup on I looked nothing like "The Lion," so I threw my head back and gave a big lion laugh. "Bah-ha-ha-ha-ha!" She smiled from ear to ear as she met the real person underneath all of that makeup.

There's a little performer in all of us. At some point or another, we can all enjoy a little extra drama. But it's nice to cycle back and show the world our true selves. I'm sure there will always be a little "Lion" inside of me and I will cherish my time with the Civic Players forever. But I enjoyed seeing the little girl smile when she saw the real me.

The acting got me far. I worked and played pretty well. I did a couple of summer plays, continued to play in a rock band, and worked for a living at the high school. I started to notice that being in plays and playing in the rock band wasn't as easy as it used to be. It became difficult to remember lines and lyrics. I would get confused recalling the information that I needed to perform in musical productions. I became frustrated because as a child, and even as a young man, I seldom forgot anything. I never wrote anything down or needed systems to help me remember. Now, I couldn't remember a damned thing. In the rock band, the lyrics and music were *always* on a stand in front of me and I would still forget things from time to time. For some reason, I started to have problems with my memory and it affected my performance.

I learned to adjust to the memory issues, though. At work I started using a "checklist." I'd never been the type to use a calendar before, but found I needed to write things down to keep them all in order. When in shows, I would record all of the music and play it while I rode to rehearsal. Since I lived in the middle of nowhere, the car ride gave me plenty of time to practice. I even recorded my lines so I could practice those. I also started using bolder fonts for printed lyrics when performing with the rock band and always printed them on one page. That made it easier to read with less possibility for mistakes if I didn't have to turn a page in the middle of a song. As technology advanced, I started putting sheet music on an electronic tablet. I developed tricks to make my life easier and help with my deteriorating memory.

So I kept on going. I kept on teaching like I'd been accustomed to. I worked all day and taught the Show Choir one night a week. Every other year we performed a musical in the fall that kept me at the school four nights a week. I played in the rock band about once a month to keep my sanity, and if I had any time left over, I spent it with Debbie. She always seemed to get the leftovers. It turned out that the leftovers were often an exhausted mess. I started slowing down and I knew it. I wondered how much longer I could continue doing things the way that I did them. Something needed to change.

14

STUCK

*W*hat makes the food in a fast food commercial look so beautiful? The hamburger bun is round and shiny. The burger is thick, juicy, and just the right color, lined up perfectly with the bun. The cheese is melted and seems to flow down the side of the burger like icing on a cake. The lettuce is a wonderful shade of green and looks like the ruffles on a tuxedo shirt. If I didn't know it was food, I'd swear it was a work of art.

Then we turn off the TV and go to the restaurant that featured that wonderful commercial. We glance up at the menu and see a picture of the same sandwich we saw on TV and it's just as beautiful. Beside the sandwich there's a picture of some French fries standing on end in a paper pouch, all parallel to one another. They look beautiful as well, all the same size and a wonderful golden brown. Enticed by the photograph, we order the sandwich and French fries and are surprised by what we receive.

Wrapped in a piece of greasy paper comes a sandwich that

looks as though it's been stepped on. It's often cold and the burger is a dry, thin disc. The cheese doesn't melt over the edge of the burger because the burger is too cold to melt it and the cheese is too small to reach the edge. The lettuce is wilted and lying in a mangled pile on top of the ensemble. The fries are cold too, undercooked, and are shoved with haste into a paper pouch. Why is there such a difference between the food on TV and the food that is served?

There's a difference between the two people who made the food. The person who made the creation on TV was an artist. He made that food, not for someone to eat, but for someone to look at. He took his time and focused on perfection. He often used paint, glue, and other things that weren't food, to make it look more desirable. The person who made the food for us to eat didn't care. He went through the motions, much like a machine on an assembly line, concerned about getting the food made, but not concerned about what it looked like. The food became part of a process instead of someone's meal.

I haven't eaten at fast food restaurants often, but have been known to ask them a question when I do. I've sometimes asked them to make mine look like the one in the picture. I would then get a blank stare and my food would come out flat and crumpled as it had in the past. In my own life I've been as stuck. I've just gone through the motions, hoping I would have the strength and stamina to make it through the day. It seems as though everyone goes through a time in their life when they have to decide whether they want to create or just survive. That's where I found myself.

So here I was, going to work every day for twenty-four years. But things had changed. I struggled getting out of bed in the morning. I struggled to put on my shoes. I worked my butt off to come up with ideas and energy to make it through a day, let alone a semester. And I hated it. Did you hear that? I *hated* it!

What happened to me? The man who once loved his job more than anything just couldn't stand to go anymore. How could I have let things get so bad? Not just for me, but for the young people that I worked with each day. The truth is, the program still thrived. There were eighty-plus kids in my classes. We still performed wonderful concerts and traveled around to different places making music. But I struggled doing it. I let things slide that I once would have *never* allowed. They may have seemed like little things to some people. There were untucked shirts during performances and students showing up late. Tennis shoes instead of dress shoes onstage. Some people might have considered those things small. But for me, they were huge. Or had been. I didn't seem to notice them anymore. I just didn't have the energy to hand paint thirty wooden canes anymore. And I didn't want to.

As a kid, I had teachers that most kids wished would hurry up and retire. They weren't bad teachers either. They were teachers who were once really good at their jobs, but over the years just lost their spark. I didn't want this to happen to me. But it wasn't my teaching ability, my attitude, my pride, or my work ethic that suffered. It was my damned health. I knew darn well that I couldn't concentrate the way I used to and I didn't have as much energy. I couldn't stay on task or create because my cycles were getting worse. My bipolar disorder had gotten the best of me. I'd worked myself into a hole and didn't know how the hell to crawl out of it. My four choirs and a guitar class were all bursting at the seams with kids. The performances we did in our rural school were still packed with people and the demands were high. How could I keep up with that while so worn down by life and health problems? I felt stuck.

The annual dinner choral revue was about a month away and I was busy creating music and choreography for that. I worked so hard to create the show that I took the wind out of my own sails. I decided to visit my doctor. Other than Debbie, few people knew that I struggled so much. I went into the doctor's office and told him the truth. "Doc, I don't know how much longer I can keep doing this. I hate it! I don't have the energy to do my job and I don't have the mania to create. I'm lost." His answer came fast. He said, "Dana, I told you to do this several years ago and now it's the time. You've got to end it. You need to quit your job." Now, I'm not the quitting type and when he mentioned this to me years ago I just laughed at him. This time I didn't laugh.

As I said, I wasn't much of a quitter so I decided to drag my way to the end of the school year even though my doctor suggested otherwise. I made the decision to leave in early March but didn't tell anyone except for my bosses. I decided that since most of the students were in my classes for several years that I would wait until the last day of school to tell them so I could exit without any kind of parade or fanfare. I continued to work every day and the fact that I would be leaving at the end of the year somehow made things go a little easier for me. I still struggled to get up each day and go to work and the ideas weren't pouring out of me the way they used to, but I knew the end was coming soon and that was a relief.

I needed to bring my decision to the administration. I talked to the superintendent about my departure. It surprised him, but I found him to be very understanding and helpful. I worked under two principals and when I talked with them, they weren't as surprised. Through the years I dealt with many health issues and though I kept them to myself as much as possible, I sometimes felt it necessary to talk with them about the challenges that made my life so difficult.

Though I never let my journey with bipolar disorder interfere with my teaching, I'm sure some of the people who worked closest with me could tell things weren't always right. There were two very close friends in the school district whom I confided in. When I made my decision to leave teaching, I talked with them about it and they became part of my support group. Being the high school choir director, I worked side by side with the band director. He and I were very close friends and still are to this day. When I told him of my decision to leave teaching he gave me his complete support. I felt bad for breaking up such a fine team. He didn't like the idea either, but had seen me through some dark times and understood. We worked together for ten years and accomplished many good things. I had a hard time walking away from that work relationship. But it didn't stop there.

My other team was even harder to face. Debbie saw me through everything in my professional life and when I made the decision to leave she gave me her complete support. She saw me struggle for several years and knew I should move on. But we still had to tell our kids. Because they were now grown children and didn't all live under the same roof, we wanted to wait until we could get them all together. We weren't sure how they were going to take the decision because a music teacher was all they'd ever known me to be. We also needed to prepare them for the idea that I wouldn't make as much money as I used to and that would affect our whole family financially. They had all witnessed my battle with bipolar for years. They saw ups, downs, and frustration. They all saw the manic episodes and lived through all kinds of turmoil. They would be prepared for the change.

My kids all came home for a weekend, so we decided to have a family dinner and break the news to them all at the same time. Family meetings were common so they weren't surprised when we sat down to have a discussion, but all of their chins hit the ground when the topic came up. After we explained it all to them they started to nod their heads and agreed that it would be the best thing. There were questions about how I would survive financially and what I would do with myself. When I responded with "I don't know," they laughed.

Nervous, scared, and even a little ashamed, it comforted me to have family support. My parents and siblings were not going to be as understanding. In twenty-four years, I hadn't done much of anything but work. Friends were close, but few. I didn't hunt or fish. I wasn't into sports. I didn't hang out with buddies at the bar. All I did was work. For nearly three decades I'd devoted myself to the school and never let my illnesses interfere with any of it. Only in the last five or six months did I find myself taking a day off a week because I needed to rest. During my last two years of teaching, I would also come home early with migraine headaches that were so painful that I needed to lie down.

Reminding myself of all of this told me that I made the right decision. I still struggled with the choice because most people work until they're at least sixty. But what else could I do? I couldn't concentrate very well anymore. Stringing words together and staying on task became a struggle. My memory issues were becoming more and more severe. While working I had three or four migraines a week. All of these issues, combined with the mood swings, were making it impossible for me to do my job. As I stated before, I had grown to hate my career, and my life, for that matter. I didn't see how I could continue. The more I thought about it, the more the decision made sense. But after twenty-four years of teaching, eighteen of them in the same small town, I wasn't sure how people were going to respond to the news.

The final day came near. The end of the school year

would soon be here and I would face my choirs and the high school staff and tell them that I would no longer be at the helm of my program. Before I had come to this town, the choral program didn't exist. There had been no vocal music in the school system whatsoever. In just a few years we'd created a remarkable program, and eighteen years later, our community started to take it for granted. They assumed that there would always be a fabulous Christmas concert and dinner choral revue, not to mention the spring show and graduation performances. Many other concerts took place throughout the year and the community showed up knowing they could count on a quality performance. At community functions such as Rotary Club, library fundraisers, Optimist Club dinners, hospital charity events, and the like, the choir would almost always be there. Now, the guy who insisted they be there was stepping down. I knew someone else could come in and take over, but I didn't know how the students would take to the idea. I found that when I stopped to think about it, I felt a little uncomfortable with it myself.

The last day of school came and I gave my final exam to the concert choir as planned. They finished with time to spare. I asked them to sit and listen to a very important announcement. I didn't tell them I was retiring, because I wasn't. At that time, I would take a medical leave of absence to improve my health, but I didn't tell them any of that.

I went on to tell them that this year would be my last year of teaching and that I would not return in the fall.

At that point, tears flowed from many of them because I'd taught them since middle school, in some cases, six years. I told them that it was a medical decision based on my health, not my feelings for them or for teaching. (I lied a little.) At that point I didn't enjoy teaching anymore, but it wasn't because of the students. My health had worn me down so far that I didn't enjoy much of anything. They asked a lot of questions about what would happen to the choir and who would take my place.

Those were all questions I couldn't answer. But I did tell them this: "When the school system finds a replacement for me and you move on with a new teacher, you'll be in a wonderful situation. You will have the opportunity to work with more than one director. That doesn't have to be a bad thing. Now, you can make it difficult by giving the new teacher a bad time, for the simple reason that he isn't me, or you can learn as much as possible and enjoy having two directors." I mustered up the best advice I could give them as I moved on to new things and they tried to move ahead with a new director in my place.

I found out the news of my leaving spread through the school and the town in a hurry. In the age of cell phones, texting, and Facebook, the kids in the choir networked my news throughout the area in less than an hour. When I went to the teacher's lounge for lunch, colleagues flocked, asking about my decision. I confirmed that I was leaving, but said very little about why. They respected my privacy and I didn't have to give many details. I never needed to play the "Bipolar Card." I still wasn't ready to let that news out. At this point I didn't know what my future entailed and I kept the details of my mental illness to myself. I was just getting used to the fact that I'd no longer be teaching music. I needed to find new things to do with my time and hoped the transition would go smoothly.

I cleaned up most of the junk that I'd accumulated over eighteen years, and left a lot of it behind as I walked out in mid June. I handed over my keys and that was that. I didn't put as much thought into that as I should have because over time, there were a lot of things I inadvertently "gave" to the school system that I would have liked back.

I feared what might happen when the school year began in the fall. I had taught for so long. It was all I knew. Although I couldn't stand my job when I left, I knew I would still miss it. That prediction proved accurate. Debbie taught in the same school system and was nowhere near retirement age, so when the school year started, she would go off to work and I would be home alone. With a long list of home projects and a new puppy to keep me company, I figured I would have plenty to keep me distracted. I was wrong about that.

15

ROLLER COASTER RIDE, MY ASS!

beautiful morning in May rolled around and my father fired up the '59 Willy's Jeep. Soon my mother, two sisters, and I climbed aboard. We went into the woods to see all of the vegetation that sprang to life on the hillsides. It rained the night before and the water glistening off of the leaves smelled fresh and wonderful as we rode along looking for just the right place to pull over and begin hunting for something special.

In the springtime in northern Michigan, after a rainfall, a little guy known as the morel mushroom will often grow in the ground and peek through the leaves waiting for someone to come along and snap it up. That was what we set out to do on this wonderful Saturday morning. We found a place to pull over and jumped out of the Jeep. We began frolicking through the woods in search of as many morel mushrooms as we could find.

I searched and searched but couldn't see the morels that were often right in front of me. My Dad would grin and say,

"Look right in front of your left hand." I'd continue looking but could not see the mushroom that my Dad assured me was right in front of my face. No matter how hard I looked, I just couldn't see the mushroom camouflaged against a field of brown leaves.

I've often wondered how many answers to questions about my life were sitting right in front of me. How many "morel mushrooms" have I walked past because I couldn't see them? If I continued to look, maybe I would find them.

My decision to leave work hit me, full throttle. The new school year came and Debbie went off to work. I stayed home. For the first time in my memory, I didn't have a job. Being a pretty industrious little kid, I'd mowed lawns, picked cherries, ran rummage sales, whatever I could do to make a buck. In my teens I went to work at a local hotel working in maintenance and later moved to the dining room. From there I worked in restaurants, bars and even drove a laundry truck. I'd never been without at least one job. As soon as I graduated, I became a teacher and worked for the next twenty-four years. While teaching, I worked nights in a hardware store and painted houses on weekends. But now, going into my fiftieth year, I would stay home. I would stay home while my wife worked. It was no big deal. I would find things to do. I wouldn't be distracted by the high school going at full tilt a scant half mile down the road.

Did you hear that? I only lived a half mile from the school, so when the marching band practiced I could hear them. I could see kids walking to school each morning and watch them come home in the afternoon. Everything about the day made me feel that I was in the wrong place. The sights, the sounds, and even the smell of the cafeteria food reminded me of the job I hated so much and I wished I could go back to! A close friend retired the same year I left. I called him to see how things were going. He said, "I'm in Virginia! I decided to get out of town for a week to make the transition into retirement easier!" What a good idea. My kids lived in different states and would have loved some company. Why didn't I think of that? But NO! I stayed home and felt sorry for myself! I whimpered and whined about the fact that everyone went back to work leaving me with nothing to do. I sat and stared at the walls while everyone went about their business. Bored and alone, I felt sorry for myself for months. At the time of this writing, it's been many years since I left teaching and I still miss being with kids.

But I soon found things to do. I got a new puppy in the spring when school let out, so I could take him for walks whenever I wanted. That gave me an idea. I started walking dogs at the animal shelter. Later I volunteered, teaching a computer class for the elderly. I sang for senior citizen luncheons once in a while and did home improvement projects when I could. The home improvement projects went pretty slow, but over time they were completed. I put new floors in much of the house and repainted rooms. I redecorated a lot of rooms and did whatever I could to stay busy.

I often dreamed about my job and wanted to go back. When I became a teacher I had power. Filled with energy and ideas, I never dreamed that it would end so soon. Sometimes I felt that fucking bipolar disorder stole my life from me! Medication made me into a goddamned zombie. It took something that I loved away from me and turned me into a different person. I frequently felt, and sometimes still feel like a stupid idiot. Other times I thought maybe a new life would come along. I just didn't know what that new life could be. I couldn't remember things. I couldn't concentrate the way I used to. Sometimes it just pissed me off!

Why the hell should I sit home and dream up a new life with new things to fill my time? The only thing I ever wanted to do was be a musician and work with kids. But bipolar disorder wore me down to the point where I hated it. It turned me into someone I didn't like anymore and made me dependent on medication. As I wrote this, I was constantly afraid I'd been making living with bipolar sound easy. It wasn't easy. I'd heard bipolar disorder described as being similar to a roller coaster ride since it has ups and downs. Blah, blah, blah. I never liked this analogy because, for the most part, roller coaster rides are FUN! Except for the occasional guy who pukes, everyone has a great time, the whole time.

Bipolar disorder is NOT a roller coaster ride. It doesn't last a minute and a half. It's miserable and it lasts forever. Bipolar takes some of the most intelligent and creative people and often pushes them to the point where they don't know if they can go on. They can't create. They can't think straight. They can't concentrate, and sometimes they can't remember. It messes with their emotional constitution in a way that has them feeling on top of the world one day and in the pits of hell the next. In addition, it continues to worsen with age so even if it's treated, it needs to be routinely revisited to keep it under control. That is what bipolar disorder did for me, but being a responsible person with a wonderful support group, I decided to kick bipolar in the ass.

I did everything my doctor told me to do. I went to neurologists and psychologists. I went to psychiatrists and scheduled MRIs, EEGs and EKGs. I took all of my medications properly. I quit drinking altogether when they told me to and saw a counselor. My blood levels were checked on a regular basis. I functioned well with medication and counseling, but I wasn't the same as I used to be. I wasn't as creative. I didn't have as much energy and I wasn't as much fun to be around. I wasn't quite a different person, but I'd changed. People who knew me well recognized it. They didn't come right out and say it, but I could see it in their eyes. I still had a sense of humor and tried to be a nice guy, but I wasn't getting drunk and jumping off of the roof anymore. Once a friend came up to me at a party and said, "You're no fun now that you don't drink anymore." I laughed with him and continued to mingle, but I knew what he meant. I thought he was an asshole for saying it, but I did know what he meant.

There's more to life than getting drunk and putting a boat in someone's swimming pool as a joke, after all. I knew that if I were to continue my life, become a productive adult, take care of myself and my family, and find this "new me" that everyone talked of, that I would have to take my medication in the proper way. So I continued to take the required dosages of all of my medication. When I went out, I drank iced tea. I became a calmer version of me and learned to adjust to that.

As far as this "new me" was concerned, I kept looking. I continued to write music at a much slower pace than in my manic days. I found it harder to create than before, but became happier with the end product when I was more selective about what I put inside of a song. I'd become kind of a "Mr. Mom" and worked hard to keep the house as nice as I could. But although I liked taking care of the household, my memory and work rate made it so that I couldn't be depended upon. I enjoyed working on carpentry type projects but got fatigued and it took me forever to complete them. As for the future, I was waiting for a lightning strike. But it didn't seem to happen. It was clear that I'd have to look for the next chapter in my life. Since teaching music is all I ever wanted to do, I had difficulty looking beyond that.

But I looked anyway, hoping that I'd find a new niche. As a youngster, interests beyond music were plentiful. Perhaps those things were waiting to be tapped into again. There's always the possibility that I was looking more at what I wanted and not at what I needed. Maybe my needs were not yet established. The music program that I left behind evolved as I worked on it. I spent years developing it. It changed as I did. I imagined that whoever I became now would evolve much in the same way. I couldn't walk out the doors of an old life which took years to create and into the doors of a new one and expect it to be complete. The new life might take as long for me to create as the last one did.

With plenty of time to try new things and meet new people, it was patience biting me in the ass. I wanted my life to be complete and fulfilling NOW. I didn't want to change anything, try anything, or develop anything. I wanted someone to smack me on the head with a magic wand and say, "This is what you'll be doing and this is how you'll do it...enjoy!" But in the back of my mind I knew better. I'd known people who worked for pyramid marketing companies for a while because they were sure they could get rich quick, or sell candles at home parties because they wanted instant success. But I always knew that if I wanted something out of life it would be work. And that's exactly what I found. Whatever I decided to do with the rest of my life wasn't going to fall into my lap. It would take time to find my new life. Sooner or later, things would even out for me and I'd find my place.

One of the biggest snags that I encountered being home at such an early age is that I was alone. At almost fifty years old, I left my job and spent all of my days alone. Most of the people I knew were working. Even though kind of a loner, I still missed being with people during the day. As three years passed, I continued to look for things to do and people to talk to. My dog got a lot of attention.

But as much as I loved my dog and I enjoyed his company, he didn't make up for the human contact at work. I'm also afraid I may have made a mistake while working. I've said this earlier, but all I did while teaching was work. That meant I didn't take a lot of time to golf, fish, go to bars, or do any of the things that would allow me to make a lot of friends to mingle with when I stopped working. I often felt isolated at home with no one to do anything with. Some of my friends retired at or around the same time I did and I could get together with them now and again, but there weren't many of them and few were in line with my age.

As I stated earlier, I did quite a bit of volunteer work and I met people through that. People who were willing to donate their time to a charity were wonderful and I enjoyed getting to know them. But I continued looking for something I could do that would allow me to be creative and productive. It just needed to be something that made me feel confident about myself without tiring me out too much or adding too much stress. To this day, I haven't really found it. But I continued to try new things. I needed to find something to occupy my time in an environment where people could enjoy me the way I was. There must be a place like that for a former "busy kid."

BIPOLAR AND KARATE

hat is normal, anyway? It's the way I started out. I got up in the morning, as did everyone else. I went to school, came home, played, did my homework, ate supper, played some more, created, went to bed and repeated the process. Life was good. As I got older, I became more and more creative and had more and more energy. Life was *really* good. Why wouldn't it be? I was talented, popular, smart, and the world lay at my feet. I didn't look at it that way, though. As a matter of fact, I thought of myself as kind of geeky. But as time went by, I found out geeky was okay and that a lot of my musician friends were just the same. So I continued on my path and became a vocal music teacher, bartender, husband, father, housekeeper, carpenter, auto-mechanic, painter, artist, repairman, and counselor all rolled up into one neat little ball. For a long time it went quite well. But after a while, I couldn't function on straight-up mania any longer and I started to crash. I struggled with symptoms of bipolar disorder, including manic episodes and depression for years. When finally diagnosed with bipolar, I learned a lot of important things that helped me in my journey.

I needed to find a doctor whom I trusted and believed in. I knew I should do what I was told, so I did. This is true when it comes to taking medication at the proper dosage. Many people with bipolar disorder either take their medication improperly, drink alcohol while taking it, or don't take it at all. I've heard many stories of family members finding medication in the trash or arguing with their bipolar sibling or mate so they'll take their medication. And I understand it. People with bipolar disorder *like* being manic. They don't *want* to take their medication because it changes the way they feel. But the truth is, it evens them out. In the long run, it'll make them a better person. It doesn't seem like it right away, and sometimes it takes months or even years to get the right combination of medications. But it's worth it. I believe everyone who struggles with bipolar disorder should put their faith in a good doctor and find a medication that helps them even out their mood cycling.

Everyone has mood cycles. They fluctuate from happy to sad and everything in between. But people who suffer from bipolar disorder experience mood cycles that are much more extreme. I once heard an interesting way to describe cycles. Bipolar mood cycles are about a hundred times more significant than an ordinary cycle. Imagine a line graph with the "normal" mood cycle being the axis. Then try to see how far away from "normal" a bipolar person's cycle would swing. The goal with medicating bipolar disorder is to bring the highs and lows closer to the axis line. In other words, they won't go as far up or down. With the right medication combination, a person can continue to be happy, sad, angry, and all other emotions, just not to the extreme where they can be damaging to life. After a lot of trial and error, that's what bipolar medication has done for me. Even though I still have mood cycles, they are not as severe as they once were and I'm able to function.

One of the reasons that evening out cycles is so difficult is because every person suffering with bipolar disorder is different. I proved this point when my "seizures" turned out to be manic episodes. No medical professional within a hundred miles of me ever saw anything like them. But my doctor kept looking for answers. He sent me to a clinic that found the problem. Each person with bipolar disorder is going to find they might have something about them that makes them unique. The length of their cycles might be quite different than someone else's. Their manic episodes may cause them frustration or anger. They might become promiscuous or spend money they shouldn't. Whatever it is that makes them unique might also make them difficult to treat. But they aren't untreatable. They just need to be open-minded and trust their medical professionals so they can find the right combination of medications.

As I just stated, bipolar people are unique individuals. They have their own wonderful creative genius rolling around inside of them. As much as they don't want to change, because medication will stifle creativity, even out cycles, and have some undesirable side effects, it will help them lead a normal life. It will also keep them in school, keep them employed, save their marriages, help them create more often, and in some cases, save their lives. After all, they're worth it!

People with bipolar disorder are often the most creative people in the world. They deserve a chance to get their lives in order. People with bipolar disorder are not alone. Many very famous artists, musicians, actors, politicians, and athletes have been diagnosed with bipolar disorder. Famous past presidents, composers, inventors, and many more have suffered with it. Throughout history, many famous figures were undiagnosed, as the disorder had not yet been identified. But descriptions of their behaviors and symptoms suggested that they were bipolar. Some of the most creative and successful people in history have suffered from the same thing. They've endured many of the same symptoms and still managed to find success.

It's a lot of work to keep bipolar disorder under control and it lasts forever. It's important to trust medical professionals and get bipolar disorder treated right away. Also, self medication is not an answer. Tobacco, alcohol, and other stimulants do not help correct it. They can make symptoms easier to deal with for a while, but not forever. The best thing to do is to listen to the advice of a good doctor. If one doesn't get helpful advice, seeking a second opinion might be smart. It's important to get bipolar disorder under control. For me, it was important to take medication and follow the advice of my doctors.

Cars and trucks! Coffee and tea! Bipolar and Karate? One thing I've noticed during my own journey with bipolar is that it's kind of like studying Karate. There's no sparring with people and breaking boards, but the way the process works is similar. When studying Karate, each time a new level is reached, a new belt is assigned. With bipolar disorder, the levels of severity increase the longer one has it, almost like Karate. I've often thought it would be nice if they awarded me with a different colored belt each time I reached a new level of severity. "It's time to increase your medication, Dana. Here's your red belt!" I don't know if that would make bipolar disorder any easier but it sure would make it a lot more fun.

It's important to remember that bipolar disorder advances or worsens with age. But that doesn't mean the outcome is bleak. It is crucial to have it treated as soon as symptoms are recognized so it can be kept under control and the patient can be comfortable. I know where I was at in my life when I was diagnosed and first started taking medication. I also know that I still have symptoms in spite of the medications I take to control it. I shudder to think what might happen if I ever decided to discontinue my medications.

In the many years that I've been controlling my illness I've seen a lot of changes within myself. Those changes have happened with medication in place. I believe that without it, I would probably be in an institution somewhere, making origami. I have a responsibility to myself and those around me to maintain my medication at the proper dosages so I can lead the most "normal" life possible. I could never be sure this combination of medications would be the last one for me. As I've said before, bipolar disorder is a journey. I listen to my body, my family, and my doctor and keep close tabs with everyone involved. After all, the people on the outside looking in see me differently than I see myself and sometimes have a better understanding of my well being than I do.

I have a solid support group in place. I've come to believe everyone needs a support system, whether they struggle with a mental illness or not. Everyone needs a friend who doesn't mind if one throws up in the backseat of their car. Everyone needs a friend who will love them no matter what they say or do. Unconditional love is hard to find. I have a big, white, fluffy friend who greets me every morning and wags his tail at me no matter what. He hugs me even if I forget to brush my teeth or if I'm crabby. He's my true friend. Though I can't say that about a lot of people, I know it's important to have them in my life. I've found that kind of love in my wife and three children as well. If I fall, they'll pick me up. If I'm depressed, they'll find a way to cheer me up. If I'm too excited, they calm me down. They watch to see if my medication levels are right. They call to check on me when I'm ill and take care of me when I need it. They love me unconditionally, just the way I love them. The truth is, that's all I ever needed.

IT'S NEVER OVER

*W*hen I was a small child, music was always inside my soul. The structure of the music, melodies and harmonies, instrumental compositions and musical aesthetics seemed to pump through my veins. As I approached adulthood I was hearing things in music that others can't. When I would repeat a song it would always be in the right key. Earworms were commonplace. If I went to bed with a song in my head, I would wake up in the morning singing the same song in the same key. I wondered if the song stayed in my brain all night. If someone played a song for me, I could hear harmonies and instrumental parts that weren't there. Even though they weren't a part of the song, I could hear them in my head. If I heard a song once, I could remember the harmonies easily and often would arrange those songs for my choirs to sing. This ability never left me. It's part of who I am and seems to strengthen as I age. I've found that many things in my life have intensified as I've grown older. Music is one of those things.

My journey with bipolar disorder is not over. Riding down hills on handmade go-karts at an early age and building boats in my teens was just part of the learning process. Juggling my time to use almost every minute in my twenties was all part of the fun. When my thirties came along, things started to change as depression began to show up. But with the help of my family, I managed to lead a very successful professional life in just twenty-four short years.

While bipolar disorder is here for keeps, I've learned to control it as much as I can. I am no longer able to do the job I found more important to me than anything, but I've reviewed my priorities and I've discovered some things. I have a wife and three children who love me more than anything and that's where most of my attention needs to be. I've got friends and interests that I've been putting on the back burner for a long time. It's time to give them some long awaited attention. But the journey with bipolar disorder never ends.

In 2015, old symptoms began to resurface. Manic episodes that were much like seizures started coming back. Mania and depression started to reappear after years of evening them out. Topamax was no longer doing the job, so my doctor decided that we would experiment with other medication possibilities. I quickly learned that changing medications was *still* a bitch. In December of 2015 I was given Geodon, which is a fairly old drug and it didn't control my manic episodes. After a long weaning process, I moved on to Latuda in May of 2016, which seemed to even me out but didn't control the episodes.

After a lot of head scratching, my doctor sent me to a neurologist to find some answers. I immediately liked him and he seemed to know exactly what to do. He put me on Lamictal as a way to control the episodes. He referred to them as "spells" because they weren't a seizure and weren't like any other manic episode he'd ever seen. At nearly the same time, my doctor told me to discontinue Latuda and suggested Vraylar as a replacement. Vraylar was a fairly new drug when I started taking it in 2016, not even a year old. It was developed to treat mixed bipolar, which seemed to describe my symptoms very well. My doctor used me as somewhat of a guinea pig for Vraylar in that he never prescribed it to a patient before.

I started taking Vraylar about a week before my daughter's wedding in July of 2016. I was terrified to go to an eleven-hour wedding ceremony while taking a new medication I hadn't tested. Almost anything could go wrong. But the time came quickly and I needed to pull myself together and prepare for a couple of long days. All of the wedding plans that were my responsibility seemed to fail. They went to hell in a handbasket, so to speak. I ordered the rehearsal dinner food for the wrong day. The bartender cancelled the morning of the wedding and I had two kegs of beer with no way to keep them cold. All of these issues added extra stress and I didn't know if Vraylar would come through for me.

It turned out to be a wonderful fit. I had enough

energy to get through long days and enough of my personality so friends would recognize me again. A major side effect, and probably the only side effect of Vraylar for me was that I became *extremely* overheated when trying to do something strenuous. This side effect did not go away, but was a small price to pay for "normality."

After a while of taking the new drug, I found I was having difficulty concentrating so my doctor prescribed Vyvanse to help with that. Debbie wasn't nudging me under the table to keep me on task in social settings anymore. She told me I was more like myself than I had been while taking any other bipolar medication.

I don't know for sure if this will be the final combination of medications in my bipolar journey, but I'm not concerned about it. I've changed medications many times and I know I can get through it if need be. I've been taking this combination of medications for five years and haven't run into any problems with dosage, side effects, or severe cycling. I still have bouts with depression and mania, but they are mild and controllable.

My support system has widened a bit. After I stopped teaching, I opened up to many of my friends about bipolar. None of them were surprised and all of them were very supportive. As time has gone by, I've been more and more open about my journey with bipolar. I've talked to friends, family, former students, and even strangers about it. Hell, I wrote a book about it! My hope is someday I'll have the courage to speak publicly about it.

Like the book title says, it is a journey. It's a long, difficult journey I deal with continuously. Sometimes I feel as though I've been punished with this damned never-ending sickness. But, I take medications on time, every day. I pace myself so I don't become stressed out or fatigued. I'm not the poster child for bipolar disorder, mostly because I have always done what the health professionals tell me. Not all people who suffer with this illness are practical, as I've tried to be. Many people who suffer from bipolar have difficulty managing it. I don't want to make it sound easy, because it's not. It's ongoing, progressive, and exhausting. It's a downright pain in the ass is what it is!

One thing I've been able to grasp over the years is that bipolar disorder is part of who I am. As time has gone by, I've learned to embrace it. I can enjoy mania when it happens and deal with depression when it gets me down. I still enjoy social interaction and have become a better friend to many people. I know in my heart I'm going to be okay. Each day is a different one. I continue to keep bipolar disorder under control. Stubbornness and self motivation kept me in the workplace seven years longer than anyone expected me to be. Doing what the doctor said kept me out of the hospital most of the time and steered me away from trouble. I'm proud of myself and the life I've led. Some things I learned along the way and some things I made up as I went along. As stated before, what I always knew and hadn't taken into account is that there can't be a top without a bottom, an in without an out, a back without a front...or an up without a down. "Down" finally came and I kicked its ass. I'm still kicking.

ACKNOWLEDGMENTS

While the author is very proud of the work he has done, it wasn't done without advice, guidance, and love. Many people came together to make this book a possibility. Photos, photo editing, manuscript editing, proofreading, support, and love were just some of the things needed to put it all together. The following people came forward with the knowledge and support that was needed to make this book a reality: Ann Blacktop MSW, Jim Burns Ph.D, Kate Conway, Michael Lehman, Nikki Messer, Tory Eisenlohr-Moul Ph.D, Linda Ransom, Kat Szmit, Don Stroup, Mary Vermeulen LMSW, Paul Wagner DO, David Wall, Deborah Wall, Michael Wall, and Erin Webb. Without their support, this book would not have been possible.

ABOUT THE AUTHOR

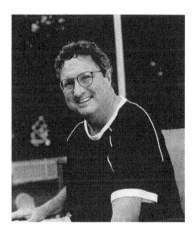

Dana Wall is a non-fiction author and former vocal music teacher from a small town in northern Michigan. His long journey with bipolar disorder, his passion for helping others, and his ability to tell a story have put him in a unique position. He has read, listened, and learned as much as he could about his illness and decided that if anyone could benefit from hearing his story then he had an obligation to tell it. He hopes you enjoy his first book. It is, after all, a book of hope. Here's to hope.

Made in the USA
Monee, IL
08 August 2022